RISK, LIABILITY AND MALPRACTICE

Commissioning Editor: Sue Hodgson
Development Editor: Nani Clansey
Project Manager: Cheryl Brant
Designer: Kirsteen Wright
Illustration Manager: Bruce Hogarth
Marketing Manager(s): Cara Jaspersen

RISK, LIABILITY AND MALPRACTICE
WHAT EVERY PLASTIC SURGEON NEEDS TO KNOW

PHIL HAECK MD

MARK GORNEY MD

ELSEVIER
SAUNDERS

ELSEVIER
SAUNDERS

ISBN: 978-1-4377-2701-2

Saunders

British Library Cataloguing in Publication Data

Risk, liability and malpractice : what every plastic surgeon needs to know.
1. Plastic surgeons–Malpractice. 2. Torts.
I. Haeck, Phil. II. Gorney, Mark.
344'.0412-dc22

Last digit is the print number: 9   8   7   6   5   4   3   2   1

CONTENTS

FOREWORD

It is an especially difficult time to be a physician in the United States. Medicine has always been a uniquely challenging profession, but for the last hundred years or so, it has attracted the best and brightest. That may be changing now as the practice of medicine undergoes transformational change, pushed by powerful forces, often in conflict with each other, directed to an uncertain point in an undefined future.

In the recent past, the practice of plastic surgery has been at least partially insulated from the economic challenges facing broader medical practice because of the widespread demand for elective cosmetic procedures that are outside the purview of most medical insurance. This has allowed the surgeon and the patient the opportunity to negotiate fees and utilization without much outside interference.

Several vectors are now acting in concert to upset that balance. First, the Great Recession has diminished the demand for elective surgery, overwhelming what had been an incoming tide of baby boomers used to unlimited horizons and seeking to maintain the appearance of their youth as they compete with subsequent generations and their own expectations for societal leadership.

Second, the elective nature of most cosmetic procedures creates a medical-legal paradox that has led to a very high frequency of malpractice litigation in the specialty. As Dr. Gorney has famously pointed out, plastic surgery is the only specialty that regularly takes well people and (temporarily) makes them sick. The parameters for successful outcomes are largely in the mind of the patient and do not readily lend themselves to objective measurement.

This is in contradistinction to most medical malpractice suits that usually pivot on the "standard of care". This concept appears straightforward enough, but it is not. The traditional notion of the standard as what similarly trained physician in the community would do under like circumstances has gradually morphed to national standards of best possible outcome achieved in ideal settings with unlimited resources. Patients unhappy with their surgeon for virtually any reason have ready access to the courts to seek redress. While most of this litigation is decided in favor of the surgeon, the process is long, exceptionally costly, uniformly unpleasant, and may, at least in some cases, have serious negative impact on the doctor's professional standing, and his/her's whole attitude toward the practice of medicine.

Third, the organizational structure of all medical practice is changing. The era of the solo practitioner and small group is ending for reasons clear enough to most in practice today. While it is clear that larger medical entities will predominate, the available models are many and it will be years before we reach a stable balance. Since plastic surgery in the community has been based almost exclusively on the solo/small group model, this conversion is often unwelcome.

In this environment of change and challenge to established pathways of care and practice, the plastic surgeon faces many hurdles. In this context, Drs. Haeck and Gorney have written a remarkable book. Written by two individuals with unique knowledge of the specialty, each chapter presents useful information not readily available elsewhere. The chapters are well arranged from those covering critical, but broad subjects ("Coping with Bad News") to very specific analyses ("The Most Risky Procedures in Plastic Surgery", "The Unique Aspects of the Male Patient and Aesthetic Surgery"). The presentation is aimed at those actively practicing the specialty and offers information and guidance integrating medical standards, cultural context, patient safety considerations, and economic grounding.

Drs. Haeck and Gorney have many decades experience reviewing malpractice litigation involving plastic surgery. They were dismayed to see many excellent colleagues succumb to poor decision making leading to years of no-win litigation. Many more claims, they found, arose from interpersonal failures between surgeon and patient. Relatively few, but these are critical, arise from intra-operative catastrophe.

The authors have undertaken the considerable labor of creating this reference for plastic surgeons in the hope of improving the clinical decision process, beginning with patient selection, offering tools for dealing with the angry patient after surgery, and sharing their long and distinguished clinical experience.

Dr. Gorney is a pillar of the plastic surgery community. He is a founding board member of The Doctors Company, the largest physician –owned medical malpractice insurer in the United States, a former president of the American Society for Plastic Surgery, the author of hundreds of scientific publications and a man who has lectured literally around the world to teach the tenants of best clinical practice of this complex and challenging specialty.

Dr. Haeck is president of the American Society of Plastic Surgery, and the author of the "on Legal Grounds" column in *Plastic Surgery News*.

He has provided expert review of hundreds of claims, and continues to practice the art and science of plastic surgery today.

Their effort is clearly dedicated to helping their colleagues make sense out of the seemingly overwhelming and daunting field of malpractice, avoiding it when possible, or when it is inevitable, living with it and seeking the best outcome with the least personal loss.

Richard Anderson
January 2011

PREFACE

In the life of a plastic surgeon, there will always be many great memories, those of success where a brilliantly executed reconstructive procedure salvaged a seemingly doomed situation, or a patient whose profuse admiration after cosmetic surgery produced deep feelings of satisfaction, even exhilaration. There may be the reflection on the first-earned payment, the reminiscences from the first office, the moment the hard-won medical degrees were finally tacked to the wall. There will be moments of positive recognition from other surgeons, feedback that meant things were going right. All these are hard to forget.

Unfortunately, there will be other types of memories as well, those that cannot be easily deleted from the memory files due to the complex emotions arising out of a single harsh moment. One of those is the precise point in time when it became apparent an unhappy patient had indeed filed a malpractice lawsuit. This will always be remembered as the start of a long journey, the one all surgeons wish to avoid traveling if at all possible.

Some have said that a malpractice case against a surgeon should be compared to a classic Greek tragedy. There will be the antagonists, the protagonists, the hero who must fight against all odds to reclaim his reputation, and evil forces hurling everything they can in the way of the surgeon to ensure the outcome will be a failure, not a victory. The story line goes through phases, or acts, and there is resolution, good or bad, to be had in the end, perhaps even a moral as well. Like the classic story, once the plot gets started, there is no way out for the hero but to continue to seek the truth. Justice must be served.

The American tort system alone is responsible for this drama. Unlike most civil courts, malpractice court is anything but mundane, stale, or monotonous. It can be dramatic, and it can often be filled with tension. Few other countries, however, insist on subjecting their physicians to jury trials. Most process medical claims through a tribunal-like system, a panel of one or more judges making the final decision, not a jury of 12 fellow citizens, virgins to the process and to medical misfortunes. Few other places in the world allow sensational amounts of money to be awarded to plaintiffs as well, no matter how egregious the claim of injury.

No one plies the trade of plastic surgery without the threat then, real or feigned, of having to go on this journey some day to face the former and now vindictive patient. Hope springs eternal but eventually the brutal reality will strike home for most surgeons. Avoiding this conflagration requires daily adherence to a set of paradigms, rules that when adhered to protect the practice, the surgeon, and the patient from calamity. Yet the rules are not neatly cataloged. There is no file on the Internet for them. Occasionally, they are discussed at risk management meetings, but that's the extent of it for most physicians. They are eventually accumulated by each surgeon over time, and personal calamity are perhaps passed on to junior partners but rarely written in one place for reference over and over.

Our intent is to change all this with a digest, a manual, if you will, for critical risk avoidance behavior. Over half of the cases we have seen headed for court could have been prevented in the first place simply through taking good care of the right patient, using sound medical judgment and reasonable record keeping. With this in mind, we set out to compile the rules, condense the conventional wisdom, and perpetuate what we have learned through our own experience with this subject over the many decades of our combined work in this arena. Our hope was to produce one single volume where our colleagues would easily find the most pertinent counsel on all matters of liability in this specialty. From consistently producing excellent informed consent to teaching the office staff some rules for handling a difficult patient, to understanding how seemingly simple cosmetic spa treatments can lead to a confrontational disaster, it is all here in one reference.

How one makes decisions in plastic surgery depends so much on the experience of the individual, the accumulated evidence of what works and what does not. It is our hope that the lessons of this book will be included in that personal space where each surgeon plies his or her trade with maximal attention to their skills, not just in surgery but also in all things having to do with patient care. Will our efforts be successful? Only time will tell. Years from now, the best measure of success for us will be the worn-down edges of these pages and the cover. By revisiting it again and again, only you the reader will determine if we accomplished what we originally set out to do.

Seattle Washington and Napa California
2011

ACKNOWLEDGMENTS

Those of us who are engaged in the difficult art of correcting deformities or improving the aesthetics of the human anatomy do so with effort, pride, and satisfaction. However, our craft also subjects us to the hot-pot of long hours of concern, anxiety, and self-reflection, a condition that places no little burden on our spouse or significant other.

It is for their continual devotion, patience, and love that both authors take this opportunity to humbly thank our two spouses, Karen Haeck and Gerri Gorney, for graciously and lovingly holding our own hands and hearts for all these many years. They are especially unique women who braved the force field of our authorship and collaboration without complaint or question.

No book could be completed without help. For their technical support and guidance we wish to gratefully thank Sue Hodgson, Nani Clansey, and Cheryl Brant at Elsevier. They saw the possibilities immediately and helped keep us on track during the many dark months of writing, never losing faith in the end product. Lastly we both wish to thank Alyson Haeck, for her long suffering transcription of large sections of our previous writing and for the keen observations she made along the way.

We are also indebted to Phil Dyer, an old friend whose knowledge of the business of insuring Plastic Surgeons was critical to helping us with the many issues of the newly burgeoning field of Medi-Spas.

Lastly, to all the employees who provided us assistance in our work for The Doctor's Company down through the years we are eternally grateful. Few Plastic Surgeons will ever understand the effort and dedication that goes on behind the scenes in this business. It is time to recognize all of them, too many to name individually, but collectively, as fine a group of smart and industrious people as one could ever meet.

Mark Gorney, M.D.
Phil Haeck, M.D.

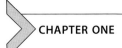

CHAPTER ONE

The Genesis of Plastic Surgery Claims

Plastic surgeons walk a fine line daily, the line that determines the direct outcome from a host of small and large decisions. Many are conscious, while many more are so routine that they rarely leave the surgeon's subconscious. All of them when combined, however, will have a direct impact on the satisfaction of both the patient and surgeon, the conclusion by both that the best outcome indeed occurred. Some of these are mega choices such as who should become a surgical patient and who should not. Many of the other choices border on minutiae, such as which layer in the closure of an incision should get which suture, or how much bleeding should be stopped immediately, and how much can be left to coagulate by itself without cauterization.

These choices come from a variety of sources, such as training, experience, recommendations of colleagues, and attendance at seminars and scientific meetings. Applying them to each unique situation encountered becomes the art of the specialty. Ignoring the consequences of the science and always "getting away with it" however can eventually overtake even the most artistic surgeon.

It is in this context then that a small group of plastic surgeons review the outcomes of their colleagues, the process of expert review of malpractice claims filed against the surgeon. Mostly these are the results of a surgery that turned out to be not so special, or rather, the patient thought it was not. At some point, for nearly every surgeon in this specialty, a patient will leave the realm of the doctor-patient relationship behind and take on the mantle of claimant or plaintiff. Once this transition occurs and a lawsuit is filed, it is up to this small group of reviewers to comment on the stages of the surgeon's decision-making, and the choices that possibly went wrong and therefore led to the unhappy ending. They are the experts that provide opinions for the lawyers, insurance representatives, and juries to consider in the future.

What went wrong and what went right in each case reviewed can be unique to the circumstances in each claim. Too often, however, a pattern

Risk, Liability and Malpractice

1

of similarity is encountered. When surgeons a continent apart, performing the same operation but on vastly different patients, are independently charged with negligence, will the root cause most likely be the same? Only a microscopic review of the elements of each case can determine that. Patterns of recurring problems, however, seem to arise, in some instances, all too often. When that is the case, the reviewer pauses to wonder. What is it that keeps bringing these cases back to the courthouse? Many can be traced back to the result of faulty decisions, large and small. Some are unique but could have been avoided with correct logic, awareness of what others would do in the same situation, or just plain old continuing education. In too many situations, knowing finally in hindsight how an adverse outcome occurred, the reviewer is left thinking, *if only this surgeon knew in advance what was going to lead to this. . .*

It is in this context that the idea for this book took shape. Knowing that there are few resources for surgeons to study and learn from the mistakes of others, it became imperative that the knowledge gained from performing thousands of claims reviews should be shared. Like a secret trunk, one that few could open, this trove of answers to what went wrong needed to be opened for all plastic surgeons to rummage through.

Each surgeon's decision pattern may be slightly different from the norm. That is clearly recognized. But what distinguishes a great surgeon from the more common variety is the ability to question and learn from a bad decision, a choice that turned out to be regrettable but not disastrous. Accepting that the old way of doing things needs to be changed, a surgeon going down this path displays a willingness to seek and adopt new paradigms. Patients win when this occurs. They lose, ultimately, when the surgeon refuses to admit that he or she needs to make new choices or simply refuses to adopt new paradigms.

When the reviewer encounters a surgeon who seems oblivious to learning from his or her mistakes, it can cause a certain poignancy, almost a malaise. Why did he or she not get it? For reasons of privacy, for medical-legal needs, it is impossible at that point to openly communicate what needs to change for that surgeon. The result of this urge is found therefore in these pages, the need to remind our colleagues of the fragile line they walk with every decision each and every day that can bring joy or angst, happiness or sorrow, glee or dejection.

The following chapters then hopefully will end the chain of errors some of us make. None of us is perfect; some of us however are just better at responding to erroneous choices. All of us need to hone the capacity to learn from mistakes.

The remainder of this chapter covers the things that all too often seem to be the source of recurrent claims in this specialty. These are the more repetitious problems, the sources of claims that crop up over and over. Their inclusion here should surprise no one in the specialty. How they lead to claims may be unique in each case but the impact of these mistakes on each surgeon will not be.

SMOKING AND NICOTINE CONSUMPTION

Studies have shown that nicotine, a potent vasoconstrictor, from various sources, can significantly compromise the capillary flow to the skin. When that skin has been lifted from its normal blood supply and then laid back in part or in whole, the resumption of a capillary network is the key to its survival. Physiologically, the stages that make a plastic surgeon look like a hero or a goat run in days here, not minutes or hours. It is this critical time phase that all plastic surgeons universally depend on for this new blood flow across the incision to achieve the best outcome. Nicotine is therefore the enemy of skin survival and it should well be considered so.

Yet cases continue to be filed over a poor outcome from surgery when the patient clearly continued to ingest nicotine despite the forewarning or even pleading by the surgeon. Some of these cases are the result of simple misunderstandings. The patient stopped smoking cigarettes but then went out and purchased nicotine gum or the trans-dermal patch. No matter where it comes from, nicotine is still the enemy of a good result and juries can be made to understand this. Explaining this in court can seem trivial but if the surgeon blames this on the patient but recorded no effort to prevent it in the chart, this excuse will seem weak and disingenuous.

Other sources of this problem occur when the surgeon failed to ask at all about nicotine usage, and the patient admits in court he or she certainly would have stopped had he or she known about the risks. Others come from out and out lying, where the patient claimed to have stopped but then "cheated" a little, unable to simply overpower his or her addiction without help. These types of cases have their own unique merits for going to a jury; some however are better off settled so that the parties can each move on. Many are simply dropped after a few years when the attorney for the patient realizes the futility of pressing on.

In an ideal world, when the patient admits to heavy nicotine use, the surgery, whether elective or not, should only take place after a specified non-ingestion period. He or she must agree to the surgeon's mandate to postpone the procedure for a minimum of two weeks, preferably one month. If necessary, surgeons should have their patients sign a document stating that they have not used nicotine for the specified period and will not use it for the same length of time postoperatively. Freely submitting then to laboratory testing can settle the matter and get to the truth. Any patient that refuses to be tested should be avoided and sent on his or her way. Operating on the nicotine user who just can't quit is a risk each surgeon must evaluate in his or her own mind, and take actions appropriately. Setting a rigid standard and sticking to it is probably still the best way to avoid the need for getting to know a defense attorney down the road.

LACK OF DOCUMENTATION

It has been said over and over again that the best defense a plastic surgeon can have is a well-constructed chart. In fact the first thing a plaintiff's attorney will do when an angry patient consults him or her is to obtain a copy of the patient's chart. When it arrives and is sloppy, missing informed consent documents for each procedure, or fails to contain key other items such as operative reports, lab values, or simple chart notes for key encounters, the odds of making this surgeon look bad in front of a jury go up. On the other hand, when the chart is in perfect order, contains the entire spectrum of documentation, and is self-explanatory of what went wrong, that attorney will have to ponder harder whether or not to accept that case.

Why then would a surgeon with great skill fail to insist on organizing great charts to reflect that? Faulty charts are not accidental. They come from a pattern in an office where little-to-no concern is paid to the matter. Hurried staff, overburdened and under-appreciated, have nothing at stake in this process. Staff that own the charting process, however, who know that mistakes can and do occasionally occur with charts and who work hard to correct them are the first line in a surgeon's defense.

While a surgeon's reputation is made among his or her patients from the surgical results, his or her inattentiveness to detail outside of the operating room will sooner or later become a potential downfall. Even the best inter-personal skills and the finest hands cannot overcome complete disorder in charting. When the disaster inevitably occurs regardless of whose fault it is, the plaintiff's attorney, not the patient, will pass judgment on the merits of the case. Why give him or her the fodder he or she needs to proceed when the claim may otherwise be greatly defensible?

While most defense attorneys claim they can always overcome a faulty chart, it is not necessarily guaranteed and will require much more effort than might have been needed to win a case. Great charts reflect great surgeons most of the time. Resolving in every patient to have the best chart possible goes a long way when that one claim arises from the least expected source.

INFORMED CONSENT

The importance of obtaining a patient's full informed consent cannot be over-emphasized. The process is so important that it will be reviewed at multiple points in this book including the basic fundamentals of correctly obtaining it.

When the patient ends his or her relationship with the plastic surgeon and goes on to become a claimant the medical reviewer or the expert witness will look at the chart for a number of important elements. It is shocking however when scanning these documents to find the number of surgeons who will proceed to an operation without the patient's signature on the chart. In too many instances, the document has been placed in the chart by office personnel, with neither the patient nor the surgeon having signed it! When it comes time to portray the surgeon in front of a jury as careless and reckless, imagine how easy it is for the plaintiff's attorney to prove this fact with a consent that went completely ignored.

When multiple procedures are scheduled, it is paramount to have each one consented to separately even though in almost all well-written consent forms there will be the phrase "and any other procedures deemed necessary by the surgeon during the operation." When the time comes for the plaintiff's attorney to list the complaints and the injuries his or her client suffered during each one, he or she will often unbundle the various parts of the surgery in an effort to prove that the patient did not consent to certain parts of what took place. For instance, most surgeons performing an abdominoplasty will also perform liposuction on the abdomen to refine the appearance and benefit the final result. When this same procedure goes to trial, the claimant will insist that they did not know that any liposuction would be performed and they certainly didn't give their consent to it.

Similarly, the various parts of a rhinoplasty increasingly are being broken down by inventive plaintiff's attorneys when the expert witness for the claimant states that, for instance, infracture wasn't needed in this case. Refuting the charge that the patient never consented to infracture becomes one more necessary step needed to defend the surgeon no matter how patently absurd it may seem. These seemingly preposterous battles, however trivial, must be fought and won, and how one performs that in front of the jury will display one's character and maturity. These battles can even work in favor of the surgeon when juries are made to see them as simply harassment from the plaintiff.

Must one therefore add needlessly superfluous wording to the consent form to ultimately defend oneself? Not in most instances. If the procedure calls for the same steps in every case and it is the standard of care for reasonable and prudent surgeons, one needs no more than the usual consent form. But when doing more than one procedure such as adding a chin implant to a rhytidectomy, the best method to completely protect oneself is to produce a second informed consent that spells out what can go wrong from augmentation genioplasty.

PATIENT SELECTION CRITERIA

Plastic surgeons' opinions vary considerably when it comes to the decision on whom to operate and whom to say no to. Increasingly common is the number of claims arising from the performance of three or more procedures on the same patient over a single ten-or-more hour anesthesia. A facelift and a breast reduction, or an abdominoplasty and then also a liposuction, can be performed safely at times on the healthiest of patients. But even they require adequate monitoring. When the patient has a Body Mass Index of over 40, is frankly obese, and has no one to care for her afterward except a teenaged daughter who is frightened out of her wits by her mother's postoperative appearance, then it is a recipe for disaster.

Patient selection will be dealt with in more detail in the following chapters as it cannot be overemphasized that this is the root cause of many malpractice claims. Successful surgery depends on doing the right operation on the right patient. When the wrong operation is done on the right person there will be dissatisfaction. But in the right or the wrong operation on the wrong patient will incur multiple problems.

Defending the surgeon's choice to operate on the wrong patient requires skill, but no matter how ingenious the defense attorney may be, the jury ultimately will become the arbiter of this. Many jurists are smart enough to ask the same question the expert witness will when first reviewing the claim: *What was the surgeon thinking?* Chapter 3 delves into the question of suitability extensively and should be considered the yardstick by which the surgeon decides whether he or she is indeed only operating on the right patients.

SCARS

It cannot be overemphasized that this specialty creates scars after virtually every surgery that its practitioners perform. While small-scar surgery such as laparoscopic procedures have caught on in other surgical branches such as general surgery and gynecology, there are only a few operations where endoscopic techniques are commonly used by plastic surgeons. In the end, there are still no broad approaches to plastic surgery that have reduced scarring.

If that is the paradigm, why not make sure that the patients are fully informed of this eventuality? They have been bombarded with the opposite, that technological advances have taken surgery into the realm of the future. But the truth is that it is still their own genetic make up that determines what the end result will be. It is much less about the surgeon's skills and more about the color of their skin, the thickness of their dermis, and the impact of infections, skin tension, and delayed healing.

Failing to tell a patient the full scope of where and how long the scar will be is all too often at the source of a claim, when other aspects of the result being told them cause high anxiety and they have reduced their comprehension. Thus when the patient feels that they have otherwise not achieved the result they wanted, and the post-surgical trade off of an ugly scar they had not bargained for intervenes, it becomes a strong motivator to seek compensation.

Defending the surgeon who adequately documented what they told the patient about the scar and all the attendant possibilities is easy. Juries do not buy that the patient forgot this conversation when it is detailed in the chart for all in the courtroom to see. If this is such a successful defensive tool, why then would a surgeon skip it nearly all the time? The fear of being too detailed and the fear of losing the patient at that point should be overpowered by the fear of having to defend the patient's claims that he or she were not fully informed. At least half of all claims against plastic surgeons will contain some sort of charge that the scar was not what the patient bargained for and that it ruined their result, affected their relationship with their spouse, and dragged down their self-esteem. It is a rare claim in this specialty that leaves this out of the list of things that the surgeon should have to pay for.

Scars and what they mean to claims are so important that they are prevalent issues in the rest of this book. Dealing with them is necessary and is the lynchpin of the surgeon's basic defense strategy.

SUMMARY

The repetitious nature of the root causes of claims in plastic surgery makes the surgeon who fails to recognize them seem distinctly out of touch. Arrogance is no substitute for knowledge. Herein lies the basis for why we chose to share our knowledge of the claims process. Our hope is that someday the specialty will be composed of surgeons skilled in anticipating what is needed to prevent claims, and, when they are unavoidable, protected themselves before they picked up the knife so that when all is said and done, they will finish their careers unblemished by the drama of a lawsuit.

CHAPTER TWO

Legal Principles Applied to Plastic and Reconstructive Surgery

Of all the medical specialists, the plastic and reconstructive surgeon's exposure to professional liability is unique in two respects at least: 1. The plastic surgeon who performs elective surgery is not assuming the care of a sick or injured patient to make him or her well. 2. Rather, it is a matter of making a healthy person temporarily sick in order to make him or her better. At that end point, the results of this treatment are judged by the patient according to standards that are entirely subjective. The actual result may be good, but if it does not meet the patient's expectations, the procedure may be judged a failure. No other specialty receives this treatment at the hands of the patient, since the gold standard for others is simply, "Did the patient get well or not?"

After years of practicing in this specialty and teaching the risks involved and evaluating claims against plastic surgeons, the authors have come to the conclusion that there are two elements critical to successful plastic surgery: patient selection criteria and truly informed consent. Nearly all the liability claims can be boiled down to these two issues, assuming that the surgery itself was without catastrophe.

This book is organized to provide insight into the multiple facets of that space where plastic surgeons and their patients grind into dissonance: the unhappy patients and their families who are no longer content to accept the final result, and the surgeon who is no longer eager to make amends.

Each chapter provides its own unique approach to the problems encountered regularly in this specialty. Whether one practices purely reconstructive surgery, purely cosmetic surgery, or as most of us do, some type of mix of the two, there is much that will pertain to everyday decision-making or the rare wrong decision.

The remainder of this chapter describes the plastic surgeon's obligation to the patient and reviews in some detail the specific principles in the surgical specialty that are the most frequent source of litigation. These fundamentals will resurface at times in the following chapters. However, to begin with, explanations of how they are important to this specialty are needed, for the obvious reason that a working knowledge of them, along with other dictums in the following chapters, helps the reader.

STANDARD OF CARE

Malpractice generally means treatment that is contrary to accepted medical standards or that produces injurious results in the patient. Most medical malpractice actions are based on laws governing negligence. Thus, the cause of action is usually the "failure" of the defendant/physician to exercise that reasonable degree of skill, learning, and care ordinarily possessed by others of the same profession in the community. Whereas in the past the term "community" was accepted geographically, it is now based on the supposition that all doctors keep up with the latest developments in their field. Community, then, is generally interpreted as a "specialty community." The standards are now those of the specialty as a whole, without regard to geographic location. This series of norms is commonly referred to as the "standard of care."

WARRANTY

The law holds that by merely engaging to render treatment, a doctor warrants that he or she has the learning and skill of the average member of that specialty and that he or she will apply that learning and skill with ordinary and reasonable care. This warranty is one of due care. It is legally implied; it need not be mentioned by the physician or the patient. However, the warranty is one of service, not cure. Thus, the doctor does not imply that the operation will be a success, or that the results will be favorable, or that he or she will not commit any medical errors as a result of a lack of skill or care.

DISCLOSURE

While attempting to define the yardstick of disclosure, the courts divide medical and surgical procedures into two categories: common procedures that incur minor or very remote serious risk (including death or serious bodily harm), for example, the administration of acetaminophen, and procedures involving serious risks for which the doctor has an "affirmative duty to disclose the potential of death or serious harm and is bound to explain in detail, the complications that might possibly occur."

Affirmative duty means that the physician is obliged to disclose risks on his or her own, without waiting for the patient to ask. The courts have long held that it is the patient, not the physician, who has the prerogative of determining what is in his/her best interests. Thus, the surgeon is legally obligated to discuss with the patient therapeutic alternatives and their particular hazards in order to provide sufficient information to determine the individual's own best interest.

How much explanation and what details to go into are dictated by a balance between the surgeon's feelings about his or her patients and the legal requirements. It is simply not possible to tell patients everything without unnecessarily dissuading them from appropriate treatment. Rather, the law holds that patients must be told the most probable of known dangers and the percentage likelihood of their occurrence. More remote risks may be disclosed in general terms, while placing them in a context of suffering from an unusual event.

Obviously, the most common complications should be explained frankly and openly, and their probability, based on the surgeon's personal experience, should also be discussed. Finally, any or all of this information is wasted unless it is documented in the patient's record. For legal purposes, if it is not in the record, it never happened!

INFORMING YOUR PATIENTS BEFORE THEY CONSENT

Over the past few decades, most medical liability carriers have experienced a significant increase in claims alleging failure to obtain a proper informed consent prior to treatment. This trend is particularly noticeable in claims against surgical specialties performing elective procedures. In fact, it is a rare claim in plastic surgery that does not contain charges of lack of informed consent, regardless of the real crux of the matter.

Informed consent means that adult patients who are capable of rational communication must be provided with sufficient information about risks, benefits, and alternatives to make an informed decision regarding a proposed course of treatment. (The same is true for "emancipated" or "self-sufficient" minor patients.) In most states, physicians have an "affirmative duty" to disclose such information. This means that they must not wait for questions from their patients; they must volunteer the information.

Without informed consent, the surgeon risks legal liability for a complication or untoward result—even if it was not caused by negligence.

The essence of this widely accepted legal doctrine is that the patient must be given all information about risks that are relevant to a meaningful decision-making process. It is the prerogative of the patient, not the physician, to determine the direction in which it is believed his or her best interests lie. Thus, reasonable familiarity with the therapeutic (and/or diagnostic) alternatives and their hazards is essential.

Do patients have the legal right to make bad judgments because they fear a possible complication? Increasingly, the courts answer affirmatively. Once the information has been fully disclosed, that aspect of the physician's obligation has been fulfilled. The weighing of risks is usually not a medical judgment but is instead reserved for the patient.

"PRUDENT PATIENT" TEST

In many states, the most important element in claims involving disputes over informed consent is the prudent patient test. The judge will inform the jury that there is no liability on the doctor's part if a prudent person in the patient's position would have accepted the treatment had he or she been adequately informed of all significant perils. Although this concept is subject to re-evaluation in hindsight, the prudent patient test becomes most meaningful where treatment is lifesaving or urgent.

This concept may also apply to simple procedures where the danger is commonly appreciated to be remote. In such cases, disclosure need not be extensive, and the prudent patient test will usually prevail.

REFUSALS

As part of medical counseling, many state laws mandate that physicians warn patients of the consequences involved with failing to heed medical advice by refusing treatment or diagnostic tests. Obviously, patients have a right to refuse. In such circumstances, it is essential that the surgeon carefully documents such refusals and their consequences and that it be verified and noted that the patient understood the consequences.

Documentation is particularly important in cases involving malignancy, where rejection of tests may impair diagnosis and refusal of treatment may lead to a fatal outcome. All such entries in the patient record should be carefully dated.

If the information presented includes percentages or other specific figures that allow the patient to compare risks, it is imperative that the figures chosen conform to the latest reliable data. Answering in court to a charge that the percentage quoted was so far off as to impede the proper decision by the patient looks bad to a jury and can be very difficult to defend, not to mention embarrassing. At times it may be more appropriate to speak in general terms if one does not know the latest percentages, or to simply tell the patient that at the next appointment the latest numbers will be produced.

CONSENT-IN-FACT AND IMPLIED CONSENT

What is the distinction between ordinary consent to treatment (consent-in-fact) and informed consent? Simply stated, the latter verifies that the patient is aware of anticipated benefits, as well as risks and alternatives to a given procedure, treatment, or test. On the other hand, proceeding with treatment of any kind without actual consent is "unlawful touching" and may therefore be considered "battery." When the patient is unable to communicate rationally, as in many emergency cases, there may be a legally implied consent to treat. The implied consent in an emergency is assumed only for the duration of the emergency.

This issue is particularly germane to injectibles such as botulinum toxins and hyaluronic acid fillers. At social gatherings where these are injected in large groups without an informed consent document, if an unfortunate complication were to develop, the battery or unlawful touching argument would constitute the basis for a plaintiff's attorney to press on theoretical grounds for a claim.

MINORS

Except in urgent situations, treating minors without consent from a parent, a legal guardian, an appropriate government agency, or a court carries a high risk of legal or even criminal charges. There are statutory exceptions, such as for an emancipated adolescent or a married minor. The surgeon who regularly treats young people should familiarize himself or herself with the existing statutory provisions in that state. In most instances, a person who is 18 years or older can consent to his or her own treatment. With the increasing requests for cosmetic treatment, at this and even younger stages of the teenage years, it behooves the surgeon to know and adhere to the correct application of his or her own state statutes. A personal stand on this issue for ethical and moral reasons is also imperative and should be freely shared with patients.

RELIGIOUS AND OTHER OBSTACLES

Occasionally, surgeons may be placed in the difficult position of being refused permission to treat or conduct diagnostic tests on the basis of a patient's religious or other beliefs. Although grave consequences may ensue, there is little that the surgeon can do in most states beyond making an intense effort to convince the patient. In some states, court intervention may be obtained. Here too, knowing the law of the state in which one practices is advisable. In all cases, the informed refusal must be carefully documented.

If a patient is either a minor on incompetent (and the parent or guardian refuses treatment), and the surgeon knows that serious consequences will ensue if appropriate tests and/or treatments are not undertaken, the surgeon's legal and moral obligations change. He or she must then resort to a court order or another appropriate governmental process in an attempt to secure surrogate consent. The participation of the hospital's legal counsel is advisable to ensure that the legal requirements applicable in that state are met.

THE SIX ELEMENTS OF INFORMED CONSENT

Where treatment is urgent (e.g., in a case of severe trauma), it may be needless and cruel to engage in extensive disclosure that could further augment existing anxieties. However, the surgeon should still inform the patient fully and completely of the treatment's risks and consequences and record such decisions. At least the following six elements of a valid informed consent should be covered with the patient and/or the family:

1. The diagnosis or suspected diagnosis
2. The nature and purpose of the proposed treatment or procedure and its anticipated benefits
3. The risks, complications, or side effects
4. The probability of success, based on the patient's condition
5. Reasonable available alternatives
6. Possible consequences if advice is not followed

In situations where the nature of the tests or treatment is purely elective, as with cosmetic surgery, the disclosure of risks and consequences may need to be expanded. Office literature can provide additional details about the procedure. In addition, an expanded discussion should take place regarding the foreseeable risks, possible untoward consequences, or unpleasant side effects associated with the procedure. This expansion is particularly necessary if the procedure is new, experimental, especially hazardous, purely for cosmetic purposes, or capable of altering sexual capacity or fertility.

DOCUMENTATION

Written verification of consent to diagnostic or therapeutic procedures is critical. A simple entry of several lines might suffice, such as: "Have discussed in detail objectives, technique and potential complications of procedure. Have also discussed location and possible appearances of scars and sources of dissatisfaction. All of the patient's questions were answered. The patient understands and accepts."

It is to be remembered, however, that in an increasing number of circumstances, laws now require the completion of specifically designed consent forms.

Studies indicate that physicians sometimes underestimate the patient's ability to understand. If the surgeon's records disclose no discussion or consent, the burden will be on the provider to demonstrate legally sufficient reasons for such absence. The more content that gets included in the recorded chart as to what the patient was told, the better. Juries have little sympathy for surgeons who briskly told the patient little-to-nothing about what they were getting into. Juries also look unfavorably on plaintiffs who remember nothing of what they were told preoperatively about risk, when they have signed extensive forms attesting that they have read the entire document, and dated it. When the surgeon's chart is robust and details what was spelled out verbally to the patient and that plenty of time and opportunity were offered to ask questions, the lack of memory is trumped by the documentation.

It is a test of the surgeon's good judgment to decide what to say to each patient and how to say it to obtain meaningful consent without frightening the patient. Astutely avoiding the use of medical terms and jargon and trying one's best to put everything into lay terms reflect common sense and good judgment. Juries will appreciate that the surgeon made the effort to get this conversation to a level that generally anyone could understand.

No permit or form will absolve the surgeon from responsibility if there is negligence; nor can a form guarantee that he or she will not be sued. Permits may vary from simple to incomprehensibly detailed. Most medical-legal authorities agree that a middle ground exists and should be sought rather than frightening the patient out of the treatment they are seeking.

A well-drafted informed consent document is proof that the surgeon tried to give the patient sufficient information on which to base an intelligent decision. Such a document, supported by a handwritten or dictated chart note entered in the patient's medical record, is often the key to a successful defense against malpractice, should the issue of consent to treatment arise.

THE THERAPEUTIC ALLIANCE

Obtaining informed consent need not be an impersonal legal requirement. When properly conducted, the process of obtaining informed consent can help establish a "therapeutic alliance" and launch or reinforce a positive doctor-patient relationship. If an unfavorable outcome occurs, that relationship can be crucial to retain patient trust.

A patient's usual psychological defense mechanism against uncertainty is to endow the doctor with omniscience in the science of medicine, and an aura of omnipotence. Weighing HOW something is said more heavily than WHAT is said, can turn an anxiety-ridden ritual into an effective claims prevention mechanism. Psychiatric literature refers to this as the "sharing of uncertainty." Rather than shattering a patient's inherent trust in the surgeon by presenting an insensitive approach, all dialogue should be sympathetic to the patient's particular concerns or tensions and should project believable reactions to an anxious and difficult situation. There is simply no better alternative to maintaining good relations.

Consider, for example, the different effects that the following two statements would have:

1. "Here is a list of complications that could occur during your treatment (operation). Please read the list and sign it."

2. "I wish I could guarantee you that there will be no problems during your treatment (operation), but that wouldn't be realistic. Sometimes there are problems that cannot be foreseen, and I want you to know about them. Please read about the possible problems, and let's talk about them, ask me anything you want."

By using the second statement, you can reduce the patient's omnipotent image of you to that of a more realistic and imperfect human being, who is sympathetically facing, and thus sharing, the same uncertainty. The implication is clear: we – you and I – are going to cooperate in doing something to your body that we hope will make you better, but you must assume some of the responsibility.

To allay anxiety, a prudent surgeon must seek to reassure the patient without creating unwarranted expectations or implying a guarantee.

Consider the different implications of these two statements:

1. "Don't worry about a thing. I've taken care of hundreds of cases like yours. You'll do just fine."
2. "Barring any unforeseen problems, I see no reason why you shouldn't do very well. I'll certainly do everything I can to help you."

If you use the first statement and the patient does not do "fine," he/she is likely to be angry with you. The second statement gently deflates the patient's fantasies to realistic proportions. This statement simultaneously reassures the patient and helps him/her to accept reality.

The therapeutic objective of informed consent should be to replace some of the patient's anxiety with a sense of his/her participation with you in the procedure. Such a sense of participation strengthens the therapeutic alliance between you and your patients. Instead of seeing each other as potential adversaries if an unfavorable or less than perfect outcome results, you and your patients are drawn closer by sharing acceptance and understanding of the shared uncertainty of clinical practice.

Nothing is guaranteed in the art and science of plastic surgery. Be it a cosmetic procedure, reconstruction of a defect of some type or a combination of the two, the patient must be properly prepared for the outcome. It is just as important as scrubbing the hands and prepping the skin. Few of us would skip the proper precautions for decontamination before surgery. Skipping important steps in developing the doctor–patient relationship can also lead to a negative outcome. Knowing how to be inclusive of all the proper stages before the surgery begins is just as critical to a plastic surgeon as carrying out the procedure itself with a flawless technique.

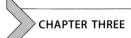

CHAPTER THREE

Recognition of the Patient Unsuitable for Plastic Surgery

Contemporary surgeons practicing plastic and reconstructive surgery in the United States will find it very difficult to end their careers unblemished by at least the threat of malpractice. The rate of claims filed against each of them was at one time as high as one claim every 2-3 years. In the period from 2005 to 2010, the rate fell as fewer claims were filed, so the average plastic surgeon can currently expect a claim to be filed once every 4-5 years. Trends always reverse themselves, so higher claim filings per year should be expected to recur at some point in the future.

Physicians who review claims against their fellow plastic surgeons feel that well over half of these are preventable. Most are based either on failures of communication or on poor patient selection criteria; few are based on technical faults. Patient selection is the ultimate inexact science. It is a mixture of surgical judgment, gut feeling, personality interaction, the surgeon's ego, and regrettably, economic considerations.

Regardless of technical ability, a surgeon who appears cold, arrogant, or insensitive is more likely to be sued than one who related at a "personal" level. Obviously, a person who is warm, sensitive, and naturally caring, with a well developed sense of humor and cordial attitude, is less likely to be the target of a malpractice claim. The ability to communicate clearly is probably the most outstanding character trait of the claims-free surgeon. Communication is the sine qua non of building a doctor-patient relationship. Unfortunately, the ability to communicate well is a personality characteristic that cannot be readily learned in adulthood. It is an integral part of the surgeon's personality. There are, however, a number of helpful guidelines.

GREAT EXPECTATIONS

There are some patients who have an unrealistic and idealized, but vague, concept of what elective surgery is going to do for them. They anticipate a major change in their lifestyle with immediate recognition of their newly acquired attractiveness. These patients obviously have an unrealistic concept of where their surgical journey is taking them and have great difficulty in accepting the fact that any major surgical procedure carries inherent risk.

Through sensitivity and communication, the smart surgeon can sense this and, once it is detected, adjust the faulty expectations of the patient or refuse to go further with any procedures. Operating on such patients carries a high risk of disappointment for all concerned. Add to this a minor complication or side effect and all types of emotional problems can surface, increasing the chance that an attorney might some day be contacted for retribution. Sending these folks on their way before it is too late makes good sense.

EXCESSIVELY DEMANDING PATIENTS

In general, the patient who brings with him or her photographs, drawings, and exact architectural specifications should be managed with great caution or refused. Such a patient has little comprehension that the surgeon is dealing with human flesh and blood; not wood or clay. This patient must be made to understand the realities of surgery, the vagaries of the healing process, and the margin of error that is a natural part of any elective procedure. Such patients show very little flexibility in accepting any failure on the part of the surgeon to deliver what was anticipated. If it is a matter of secondary repair, the odds against you grow significantly.

Some patients are increasingly prone to bringing downloaded "before" and "after" photos from the internet to their initial consultations with the new surgeon. It is imperative that seeking out the demanding, and therefore, ill-suited patient becomes an accurate exercise on the part of the surgeon. When these people are reminded that the body frames of the patients they have selected are far different than their own, and they persist and seem in denial of this fact, it should serve as a red flag for the surgeon. If this behavior continues and becomes excessive, and especially if the patient demands to know what the surgeon thinks of the results in dozens of such photos, there most likely is a good chance that this patient is not yet ready for the reality of an operation, and certainly not the anxiety of a complication.

THE INDECISIVE PATIENT

To the question "Doctor, do you think I ought to have this done?" the prudent surgeon should respond, "This is a decision which I cannot make for you. It is one you have to make yourself. I can tell you what

I think we can achieve, but if you have any doubt whatsoever, I recommend strongly that you think about it carefully before deciding whether or not to accept the risks which I have discussed with you." The more the decision to undergo surgery is motivated from within and not "sold," the less likely that recrimination will follow an unfavorable result. Patients who call back repeatedly to ask this same question or reschedule their surgery over and over again should not be considered as good candidates for any elective surgery. When they do go forward, there may be a high chance that any result will be seen as unsatisfactory.

THE IMMATURE PATIENT

The experienced surgeon should assess not only the physical, but also the emotional maturity of the patient. The youthful or immature patient (age has no relationship to maturity) usually has excessively romantic expectations and a highly unrealistic concept of what the surgery will achieve. Often when confronted with the mirror postoperatively, they are prone to react in disconcerting or even violent fashion if the degree of change achieved does not coincide with their pre-conceived notions. Avoiding this type of catastrophe requires sensitivity and the ability to simply say no, regardless of the financial implications.

THE SECRETIVE PATIENT

Certain patients who wish to convert their surgery into a "secret" and request elaborate precautions to prevent anyone from knowing that they are having anything done will occasionally surface in all plastic surgery practices. Apart from the fact that such arrangements for secrecy are difficult to achieve, this demand is a strong indication that the patient has a degree of guilt about the procedure. Thus, there is a higher likelihood of subsequent dissatisfaction. They will be acutely troubled when delayed bruising, healing, and scarring mean that their secret must be prolonged. Hiding to excess the "not yet ready for prime time" surgical results will require so much emotional effort for them that they will shift all blame onto the surgeon. Once this occurs, the staff of the surgeon will be tired of this foolishness and also shift the blame on him or her. Nothing good ever comes out of these situations except a resolution to avoid such patients in the future.

FAMILIAL DISAPPROVAL

It is far more comfortable, although not essential, if the immediate family approves of the surgery being sought, particularly in the case of a minor. When the surgery proceeds despite this, and less than optimal results occur, there will be a tendency on the part of the family to automatically react with "See, I told you so!" This can produce a secondary reaction on the part of the patient toward the surgeon, a transference of misplaced guilt and shame. The doctor–patient relationship can only suffer when this happens. Surgeons have just two choices at this point, working with the family and inviting them into this relationship or giving up on the patient, a choice that can only deepen the guilt and dissatisfaction of the patient. At this point, recrimination can rear its ugly head as the patient seeks to assuage his/her feelings. Better not to have operated than to discover, too late, that this was a poor candidate for any procedure.

PATIENTS YOU DO NOT LIKE (OR WHO DO NOT LIKE YOU)

Regardless of the surgeon's personality, in life there are people whom you simply "do not like" or who do not like you. Most experienced surgeons know within minutes of the patient entering the examining room whether they will or will not be operating on that patient. Accepting a patient for whom you feel a basic dislike (you do not need a reason!) is a serious mistake. A clash of personalities for whatever cause is bound to affect the outcome of the case, regardless of the actual quality or the postoperative result. No matter how "interesting" such a case may appear, it is far better to simply decline the patient's request. Sympathy for their plight does not necessarily mean that one must change one's rules or relax one's standards. If they seem to be somewhat pathetic in the initial examination, they will seem positively wretched when the complication occurs. These relationships can often deteriorate quickly when even small amounts of stress creep into their lives.

THE "SURGIHOLIC"

A patient who has had a variety of plastic surgery procedures performed, and who might be termed a "surgiholic," often may be attempting to compensate for a poor self-image with repeated surgeries. In addition to the implications of such a personality pattern, the surgeon is also confronted with a more difficult anatomical situation because of the variety of scars left by the previous surgeons. He or she also risks unfavorable comparison with previous surgeons. Often the percentage of achievable improvement is not worth the risk of the procedure.

Generally speaking, there is a clear risk/benefit ratio to every surgical procedure. If the risk/benefit ratio is favorable, the surgery can be encouraged and has a high probability of success. If the risk/benefit ratio is unfavorable, not only does the reverse apply, but the unintended consequences of the unfavorable outcome may turn out to be disproportionate to the surgical result. The only way to avoid this debacle is to learn how to distinguish those patients whose body image and personality characteristics make them unsuitable for the surgery that they seek, and firmly refuse.

BODY DYSMORPHIC DISORDER

As the popularity of cosmetic surgery increases, the number of patients finding comfort and solace in repetitive elective surgical procedures is growing. Are they addicted to plastic surgery? Are they surgiholics? Do they fall into a category where their unrealistic expectations for what little change will occur satisfies something other than the need to look better or simply different?

Many well-adjusted, normally satisfied cosmetic surgery patients will make a conscious decision to try something else if the first surgery was far easier than they had anticipated and recovery was a snap. Once they get their feet wet and they do not freeze to death, they will plunge into the waters with gusto. Many patients have more than one feature that they are dissatisfied with. But these are patients who are grateful for their new appearance; they seldom question the end result and they go on with their lives feeling rejuvenated and fulfilled. They are not addicted and do not have severe psychological problems masked by their desire for additional procedures.

When the physical change sought through surgery is usually more a manifestation of a seriously flawed body image than a measurable deviation from physical normality, the possibility exists of a diagnosis of Body Dysmorphic Disorder (BDD). This serious characterologic problem represents a pathological preoccupation by the patient over a physical trait that may be seen as normal by others, including a plastic surgeon. When the patient has no self-imposed limits on the lengths he/she will go to pursue surgery for a seemingly insignificant flaw, it should serve as a warning that this is not a good surgical patient.

A dead giveaway that this is the diagnosis in a new patient is the long list of other surgeons who have operated on him/her but "failed" in the patient's opinion. Heaping praise on your reputation and attesting that only you can "fix" the problems others have created in their lives is another sure sign of this diagnosis.

These patients make for many problems in the life of the surgeon, especially when in the surgeon's eyes the procedure was a complete success. This type of patient will belittle the result, question why it was performed in the way it was, and complain bitterly of the surgeon's incompetence. They distort the surgical reality and will drive both the surgeon and his or her staff to insanity with their constant calls, return visits, and complaints. Surgeons who fall into this trap often rue the day they met the patient, and seek multiple ways to refer this type out of their practice. The good news is that to continue their deception that nothing is wrong with their psyche, this type of patient does not often pursue legal action, as exposure of their mental condition might go along with the intrusions associated with depositions and trials. The bad news is that they will not stop maligning one's reputation to every other surgeon they see. Once the surgeon lays a hand on the person with BDD, his or her signature will go along with that patient forever.

PATIENTS FRIGHTENED BY THE WORD "SCAR"

Most surgeons assume that the patient understands that healing entails formation of a scar. Many patients do not even think about it if the surgeon does not talk about it. Unfortunately, for many surgeons it is seldom discussed in the preop consultation or touched on only briefly. In cosmetic as well as reconstructive cases, the appearance of the resulting scar(s) can be *the* major genesis of dissatisfaction. It is imperative that the plastic surgeon obtains from the patients clear evidence of their comprehension that without a scar, there is no healing. Without an incision there will be no scar, but in fact, without an incision, their appearance will not change.

If at this point the patient is no longer tracking the conversation, the wise surgeon steps back and investigates the reaction to the word "scar." There is little point in going forward when this has become the deal breaker for the patient. The emotional reaction to this inevitable end result can tell the surgeon that this person is not yet ready for the trade-offs that the surgery entails. Minimizing the situation at this point will only delay the inevitable reaction later when the bandages come off for the first time. The goal for that moment is to have "oohs and ahs," and not shrieking and crying.

For the patient with traumatic scars from previous emergency surgery, orthopedic surgery for fracture reduction, or cancer surgery, the consultation for "scar removal" can be a very emotional ordeal. Plastic surgeons have garnered a reputation for having the ability to make scars disappear. While scars can be improved by surgeons in this specialty, many patients make the assumption that the end result will be complete removal, once and for all, of the visible reminder of a traumatic event. When they must confront the truth with the surgeon, buried emotions over the long-standing issues these scars entail can boil over, making both the patient and the surgeon uncomfortable. Once again, in this situation, giving them hope but without diminishing the fact that there will still be a scar is of paramount importance. Promising complete removal will only lead to an angry patient when the now-improved but still-present scar is the end result they were not prepared for. These patients should be encouraged to think things over and come back for a second discussion as the emotions involved with learning the truth can overcome their ability to hear any more details from the surgeon, especially if the recommended surgery is complex, needs multiple procedures, and will be expensive.

THE ANGRY PATIENT

Patients feel both anxious and bewildered when elective surgery does not go smoothly or the result fails to meet their expectations. The borderline between anxiety and anger is tenuous, and the conversion factor from one to the other is rooted in uncertainty and fear of the unknown. A patient frightened by a postoperative complication or uncertain about the future may reason: "If it is the doctor's fault, then the responsibility for correction falls on the doctor."

The patient's perceptions may clash with the physician's anxieties, insecurities, and wounded pride. The patient blames the physician, who in turn becomes defensive. At this delicate juncture, the physician's reaction can set in motion a chain reaction, one that can lead to litigation if not dealt with smoothly and with grace and skill. The physician must learn to put aside feelings of disappointment, anxiety, defensiveness, and hostility and understand that he or she is probably dealing with a frightened patient who is using anger to gain control. The patient's perception is that the physician will understand the uncertainty of the future, and will join him/her to help overcome it. When the opposite, abandonment, occurs, this can be the deciding factor in losing the therapeutic doctor-patient relationship and act as a catalyst to promote more conflict.

One of the worst errors in dealing with angry or dissatisfied patients is to try to avoid them. It is necessary to actively participate in the process rather than attempting to avoid the issue. To do otherwise is guaranteed to stimulate a visit to the lawyer. If this conflict stirs up long-standing emotional conflicts internally for the surgeon, then getting professional help immediately can go a long way to learning how to resolve the dissonance this patient has dredged up, and can help to avoid further loss of touch with them.

Most of the litigation seen in plastic surgery has a common denominator of poor communication. The doctor-patient relationship during anxious moments can be shattered by a surgeon's arrogance, hostility, coldness (real or imagined), or simply by the fact that "he or she did not care." There are only two ways to avoid such a debacle: (1) make sure that the patient has no reason to feel that way, and (2) avoid the patient in the first place who is going to feel that way no matter what the surgeon may have done.

Although the doctor's skill, reputation, and other intangible factors contribute to a patient's sense of confidence, rapport between the patient and the surgeon, based on forthright and accurate communication, is an absolute necessity. This will normally prevent the vicious cycle of disappointment, anger, and frustration for the patient, and reactive hostility, defensiveness, and arrogance from the doctor, a series of events that almost certainly can lead to and provoke a lawsuit.

SUMMARY

In the best of all possible worlds, the prospective patient would project from the mind onto a screen exactly the changes he or she conceives, for the surgeon to decide whether or not he/she can translate that image into reality. Lamentably, we are still many decades short of achieving such imaginary technology. It is still too easy for the well-meaning surgeon to be deceived about a patient's pathological motivation. It is also conceivable that a certain physical deformity really *is* the center of the patient's psychological fragility. There are many examples of beneficial change wrought through successful aesthetic corrective surgery. Nonetheless, statistically the odds for an unfavorable result and a claim are much greater when the objective deformity and the distress it creates in the patient are out of proportion. The surgeon is cautioned to search for appropriate psychological balance and lean strongly against surgery in those cases where there is doubt.

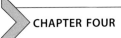
The Most Risky Procedures in Plastic Surgery

As a specialty, plastic surgery is known for innovation and perpetual dissemination of educational knowledge. Whether it is surgical permutations that enhance results or the introduction of completely new instrumentation or procedures, the advancement of the specialty is driven by information sharing. More than any of the other branches of medicine, this specialty has depended on the use of visual media and digital technology to set new standards for its practitioners. Despite this tendency toward large-scale knowledge sharing, however, there has never been an attempt to circulate to a large extent information regarding the questions of malpractice data in plastic surgery. Curiously, for a specialty that must deal with a high frequency of lawsuits and claims made against its practitioners, the unavailability of hard data that might help plastic surgeons avoid these situations is glaring.

Among malpractice liability insurance carriers, the reputation of the specialty is known for its "high frequency but low severity" risk. The frequency issue is explained on the basis of steady numbers of patients who are simply dissatisfied with their results or simply their surgical scars. Less often, the complaint revolves around frank complications. Yet when these complaints become lawsuits, the surgeons win the vast majority that go on to trial. If they lose, the severity of the verdict is usually low compared to specialties such as neurosurgery or obstetrics.

In essence however the reality and the hard data behind this axiom have essentially never been explained to the everyday practitioner in a procedure-by-procedure format. This knowledge, if available, could be useful to predict which patients might need extra-careful attention because they fall into a category where the chances are higher that they will be more likely to file a claim for malpractice if things do not work out they way they hoped for in the end.

The internet has become the prime source for information sharing in this specialty with "on-line" versions of books and journals rapidly becoming the most popular choice for advancing one's knowledge base. But using search engines to find useful malpractice data is still a frustrating venture. Beyond very large and private verdict databases used by the plaintiff's bar, very little has ever been released about these data for either public consumption or that of the surgeon. Is this because the insurers, the surgeons or the lawyers wish to keep what they know under wraps? To some extent this may be true. But is it more likely that no one ever asked? To some extent that may be so. But the truth of the matter is that there has never been a well-developed way to evaluate the data, examine them for trends, reveal where the true risk lies, and spread facts and not innuendo.

This chapter therefore addresses this situation, delineating a data study on this issue that may be far less intuitive to both surgeons and attorneys than one might think. Some of the results are expected, others surprising but explainable when the issues are researched and causes determined for spikes in claims that were not well recognized before now.

"The Doctor's Company" (TDC), a malpractice insurance company in existence since 1975, and originating from the malpractice coverage crisis of that same year in California, continues to be the largest single insurer of plastic surgeons in the United States. One in five members of the American Society of Plastic Surgeons buys his or her liability insurance from this firm. For this book, the company agreed to openly share its data taken from its experience with American Society of Plastic Surgeons member surgeons located in over 45 states. To date, this type of data sharing has not been published widely nor shared in general outside of the industry.

It should come as no surprise to the average plastic surgeon that the frequency of claims made for negligence is trending lower. What is surprising is that this trend has lasted now for almost 5 years. The old adage, that once in every 2-3 years the average plastic surgeon was named a party to a lawsuit, has been replaced with a rate drifting down to once in every 5-6 years.

While there are many explanations including the fact that the majority of states have now passed some sort of tort reform based on various caps, it is also true that the high cost of taking a plaintiff's case through 3-5 years of prolonged litigation has made attorneys more selective, especially considering the odds that plastic surgeons prevail at trial 80% of the time. In general, where a patient whose simple dissatisfaction with the results of plastic surgery (but without obvious negligence) would still generate an attorney's interest in hopes of making a quick, moderate settlement, the costs of that litigation has skyrocketed over the last ten years. This is the most likely reason that frivolous claims were filed in higher numbers in the past than they are seen today.

From 2005 to 2009, TDC has experienced between 232 to 252 claims filed for insured plastic surgeons, with a stable average of 244. Since there are just over 6,000 active board certified plastic surgeons in the United States, extrapolating this rate to all surgeons in the specialty would suggest that a total of 1200 filings for malpractice claims occur per year for all plastic surgeons in the United States. These are the derivative data that suggests one out of five to six surgeons is subject to a suit per year.

The American Society of Plastic Surgery, the oldest and largest association in the specialty, annually accumulates a wealth of information on the types and frequencies of procedures its members perform both in cosmetic and reconstructive surgery. Each year, these data are methodically analyzed and verified, and then released to the media and the public. Reporters throughout the media have become more and more fascinated, even mesmerized by the year-over-year trends that these data portray, such as "breast augmentations up 7% while liposuction cases down 4%."

Yet beyond the huge interest that this generates in the lay press, member surgeons themselves do not seem in general to be able to find specific applications for this annual binge on data. The general usefulness as a benchmarking tool for comparing one's own year-over-year statistical differences is the limit to which plastic surgeons seem to find utility with this.

To date, no one has attempted to take these two data sources and juxtapose them in an attempt to answer some important questions about high-risk cases in plastic surgery. Yet when this is done, the answers are surprising, a rank ordering of cases in the specialty that generate the highest risk, regardless of their rank in frequency.

METHODOLOGY

2007 was the year in which the ASPS recorded the highest "Procedural Statistics" in terms of the volume of procedures performed in the specialty prior to the global recession, which started in late 2008. The case volume numbers have dropped for 2008 and 2009 for cosmetic procedures. The decision was made therefore to utilize the data from 2007 as the benchmark point so as to avoid any confounding conclusions from a recession-related slow down in volume in subsequent years (Figure 4.1).

The second point in development of these calculations is that the claims data from TDC should not coincide directly with the year in which the procedural numbers occurred. Given that it takes 1-2 years after the

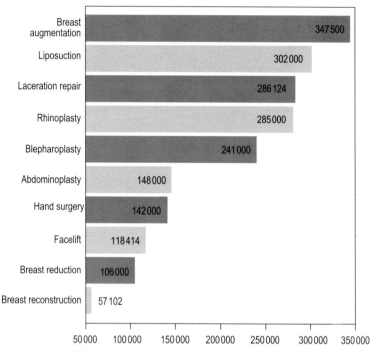

Figure 4.1 2007 ASPS most common procedures

procedure was performed for a distressed patient to find an attorney and then file a claim against the surgeon, the more likely year for making an accurate analysis of the data would be the 2008 claims numbers. The last assumption was that rates of claims for each type of procedure would be common to all malpractice carriers, that is, a similar experience to that of TDC. Given the fact that one in five plastic surgeons buys coverage from TDC, the raw data for all claims in the country were an extrapolation of the TDC claims data multiplied therefore by a factor of five. This assumes that all malpractice carriers have a similar claims experience with plastic surgeons. The argument that these numbers may not reflect the risk for every carrier is deflected by the great stability in claims numbers for the TDC experience from 2005 to 2009, essentially no change from year to year. Had TDC been able to show a reduction in claims for that same time period by introducing new risk management courses or some other educational component, this could have been reflected in the raw data. But the fact of the matter is that this period of stability in the insurance market for plastic surgery is not confined to one company.

The two categories that represent the most frequent procedures performed in the specialty are tumor removal and cosmetic injections. The numbers of claims filed over these high frequency encounters with patients in plastic surgery are small but not nonexistent. Chapter 12 deals with the risk associated with cosmetic injections, a new and very real problem, but for purposes of this chapter anything that did not require a surgical prep was eliminated. Likewise, removal of everything from nevi to cancers is in a category of its own, extremely broad but not without risk, most claims being filed in this category for failure to diagnose or incomplete removal. In the end, only the full surgical procedures are included in this research (Figure 4.2).

The calculations leading to a "Risk Index" were made by dividing the raw numbers of nationwide claims by the frequency of the number of procedures performed from the ASPS procedural statistics. This leads to a percentage ratio, the Risk Index. This number represents then a scale on which these common procedures fall and how likely the surgeon is to encounter a claim from each category. For the first time ever, it delineates which surgery is more risky rather than which claims are more widely encountered.

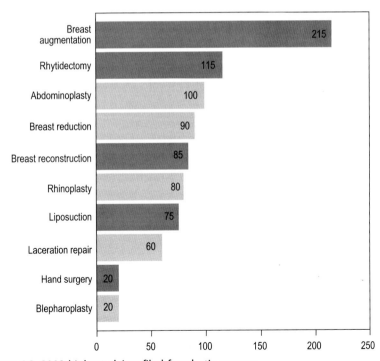

Figure 4.2 2008 highest claims filed for plastic surgery

RESULTS

Given that breast augmentation was the most frequently performed cosmetic surgery in 2007, one might have expected it to have the same rank in malpractice claims. But adjusted and indexed for claims risk, this procedure falls however to fifth place on the scale. In fact, breast reconstruction instead ranks first, despite the fact that breast augmentation is performed six times more often. The revelation is that the two procedures, although having something in common, have outcomes that are quite different in terms of patient satisfaction, complications, and overall success. A surgeon performing breast reconstruction with an implant is more than twice as likely to be named in a claim for the results than if he or she performs breast augmentation not reconstruction with the same or similar implants (Table 4.1).

The procedures that ranked lowest on the scale might also surprise many surgeons. While rhytidectomies rank very high at number two on the risk index, blepharoplasty ranks second to last. These two surgeries are the procedures most often combined in facial cosmetic surgery but now show surprisingly different risk profiles when it comes to malpractice.

Table 4.1 The 10 most common procedures in 2007 ranked by the risk index ratio and therefore the assumed risk of leading to a malpractice claim

Risk rank	Procedure	2007 ASPS raw data	2007 ASPS rank	2008 TDC claims volume	Risk index
1.	Breast reconstruction	57,102	10	85	.148
2.	Rhytidectomy	118,414	8	115	.097
3.	Breast reduction	106,000	9	90	.084
4.	Abdominoplasty	148,000	7	100	.067
5.	Breast augmentation	347,500	1	215	.061
6.	Rhinoplasty	285,000	3	80	.028
7.	Liposuction	302,000	2	75	.024
8.	Laceration repair	286,124	4	60	.020
9.	Hand surgery	142,000	6	20	.014
10.	Blepharoplasty	241,000	5	20	.008

What follows is a procedure-by-procedure analysis of the more common reasons seen by malpractice insurance carriers for these surgeries and in rank order.

Breast reconstruction

While there are many reasons why claims are filed for this operation in increasing numbers, two reasons continue to stand out. The first relates to the nature of the tissues on the chest wall after the initial extirpation. The unique challenges posed in making a soft, mobile, and realistic looking breast when most of the original tissue is missing and essentially replaced by poorly vascularized scars continue to vex even the most experienced surgeons. The second reason relates to the fact that when things go bad postoperatively, patients are prone to resort to accusations that they should have had an alternative surgery, the one they assume would not have resulted in the disaster they experienced.

The expectations for a miracle are often high with this surgery, the emotional component of breast cancer fueling a desire to get back that which was taken away, along with the desire to remove any reminders of the cancer that interrupted one's life. The plastic surgeon dealing with these situations daily or weekly will have experienced the full spectrum of the strain imposed on both the patient's tissues and psyche. The key is knowing which procedure will work for which patient. The experienced surgeon, one who performs these procedures regularly, will know when to accomplish something simple, and when to attempt something truly complex.

Often however the typical claim for breast reconstruction that did not meet the patient's expectations came about when the surgeon did not perform this surgery on a regular basis, possibly less than even a few times a year. Perhaps, the judgment in these situations was lacking, or the patient's own inherent tissue problems were not appreciated. But the bottom line is that ultra thin mastectomy flaps that have been irradiated are no place for the meek or those in a hurry. When the problems mount, such as infections, tissue loss, and implant exposures, the priority is getting the patient through the complications, and then giving hope that more can be accomplished. Some patients will quit of their own accord at this point.

With every failed attempt at reconstruction, whether it is by tissue expansion and implants or autologous tissue transfer, when the outcome is bad and the patient resorts to a malpractice claim, there is one underlying theme that is common to all these situations. That is, the patient will assert that she should have been told about the alternative operation, especially the one she was not offered. If she had a TRAM flap fail and the next surgeon successfully reconstructed her with tissue expansion, one part of the lawsuit she will file is for failure to adequately inform her right from the start that the simpler operation was even a choice. Likewise, when a second surgeon salvages a dismal failure from implant reconstruction with autologous tissue transfer, the patient in this instance will also claim being given no information about the alternatives, the operation she is convinced, was simpler, faster, and would have avoided complications she experienced.

Blame for this possibly stems from surgeon preferences, when the entire spectrum of reconstructive possibilities is glossed over to make the choice limited to the operation the surgeon wants for this patient. Or blame it on the emotional state of the patient, suffering from the stress of the diagnosis and dealing with denial, and most likely able to recall little from the preoperative discussions of the alternatives. But the overwhelmingly common theme when patients pursue lawsuits over breast reconstruction is this: "Now that I have suffered so much, had I known more about the advantages of (the alternative procedure) I would have chosen it first."

The lessons to be learned from this are many. Documentation that the patient was completely informed of the pros and cons of every type of alternative reconstruction and that she was given the ability to make her own choice based on adequate information is a must. This includes not just a signed informed consent document but also a hearty chart note describing this frank discussion, preferably dictated and always complete.

Finally, every plastic surgeon must resist the temptation to be a hero when the patient's chest wall will just not support a heroic operation. Surgeons need to respect the fact that the blood supply to the skin after reconstruction is usually insulted, and the operation chosen either will or will not re-establish this. In the end all of the infections, skin and fat necrosis and abject flap failures as well as failed tissue expansion and extruding implants relate to this concept in the majority of claims that result from these operations.

Rhytidectomy

Of the many reasons that this operation is high on the list is that when things go bad they are always difficult for the patient to hide. Breast and abdominal operations that fail can be covered in clothing. Facial imperfections cannot easily be disguised. While hair styles and make-up will go a long way to deal with some of these problems, in the end the disappointed patient will still have to confront what he or she sees in the mirror every day, and then decide how to cover it enough that he or she can venture out in public. Is it any wonder then that these claims get filed more often than any other facial operation?

Scarring of all kinds seems to be the primary reason for this. This includes visible scars around the ears and the hairline, as well as skin scars from delayed healing and tissue that was tightened beyond the ability of the blood supply to support it.

Asymmetrical ears, eyebrows, and neck account for some of the claims, but over and above the little things, the primary reason these claims get filed is the overwhelming feeling these patients have of emotional distress and their disappointment with the results, some of it unfounded and some of it clearly a result of misdirected surgery.

How does this occur? Were they really the right patients for the procedure? Over-promising and under-delivering seems to be one source. Failing to achieve the results may have just been due to the fact that the surgeon performed the operation correctly but had not prepped the patient for what was possible in the end and what was not.

In rhytidectomies, each patient must be told frankly about hematomas, infections, skin necrosis, severe scars, and facial nerve injuries. The seeds to the best defense of these claims must be sown with a thorough discussion of the possibility for a poor outcome, and then well documented for this strategy to successfully protect the surgeon at the courthouse some day.

Finally, it seems some plastic surgeons just do not know when to say no and turn a patient down for this operation. No matter how the surgeon does the procedure, no matter what little intraoperative tricks are used, the patient with faulty expectations will not be mollified easily, especially when a complication or a side effect interrupted the healing process.

Breast reduction

At the top of the list for disappointment with the results of this operation are scars. Darkened, hypertrophic, and asymmetrical, they are an embarrassment, no matter how much the patient was informed about them and their ultimate location. Dismissing the patient at this point without an attempt to improve the situation does not score any points. While few of these lawsuits are won in court, the surgeon will be preoccupied with the defense of it for years. Avoiding this situation involves adequate patient preparation, as well as careful patient selection in the first place.

Patients whose ethnicity will leave them prone to scar hypertrophy or keloids need more than just a passing discussion of the potential for this to occur. The worst choice for the surgeon is to have no discussion at all about the potential for uncontrolled scarring.

Secondary to the scar issues comes the incident with major tissue loss and a subsequent disastrous appearance of one or both breasts. A breakdown in the blood supply to the pedicle with nipple loss, skin flap necrosis, and dehiscence with a subsequent infection will leave most patients feeling deformed and cheated. Serial photographs taken by them of this calamity can impress a jury. The failure of the surgeon to reverse the disastrous results of the operation early on can lead a jury to sympathize with the distressed the plaintiff. The defense strategy that this complication was not the surgeon's fault and the patient was aware that it could happen to anyone including her also goes over poorly with most juries. Winning these claims is very possible if the patient was a nicotine user and was told to quit preoperatively, but did not. In the end, some of these claims are successfully defended despite the visual impact the scars will have on the jury because the surgeon had fully documented that they had well prepared the patient for this eventuality, tried hard to get the best result in the end, and impressed the jury with their sincerity.

Abdominoplasty

The ways in which this operation leads to a malpractice claim are multiple. Many relate to midline tissue loss, with resultant scarring and disappointing visual results. Some result from deep venous thrombosis, pulmonary embolism, and the associated high costs of the resultant therapy. But what has become increasingly problematic is the combination of an abdominoplasty and one, two, or three other major operations, all performed during one prolonged anesthesia session, sometimes lasting up to 10 or more hours. When these patients are discharged to their homes with a naïve caregiver, poor instructions, and a heavy load of medications, the occasional disaster will inevitably occur. When they have a BMI of 35 to 40 and higher the motivation of the surgeon will be questioned, since common surgical sense appears to have been abandoned in these instances.

The underlying theme to these cases is usually poor patient selection. A physically fit woman who exercises regularly can undergo this combination of procedures with a modest increase in risk from blood loss and prolonged anesthesia. But a woman with a high BMI and a sedentary lifestyle will be physically challenged much more by this combination, especially if there are significant complications of any kind.

Sending healthy patients home after this operation is in itself not necessarily a problem. Admitting them to a recovery center will also not prevent a complication from occurring. But wrongly anticipating who needs just a little TLC and who will need full monitoring seems to be the misadventure most often linked to catastrophic problems after surgery of this complexity.

Breast augmentation

While this operation ranks as the number one surgical procedure performed by plastic surgeons in 2007 and is the most frequent source of claims for plastic surgeons in 2008, when it is ranked by the risk index methodology, it falls towards the halfway point on this list. Some surgeons will be surprised by this, while others will understand that the high frequency of women asking for this procedure is not the crux of the problem. The fact is that few of the claims from augmentations are derived from a single operation.

The key to understanding why claims get filed for this operation lies in the fact that one out of three women who have an augmentation will have at least one other operation within the subsequent 5 years or less. The common theme that runs throughout the claims for this surgery is that nearly every woman who files suit for dissatisfaction with her breast surgery has had at least three or more surgeries. Some have had six or more. Another way to look at this is the fact that for every two women who have a pleasing result from this operation and are satisfied right from the start, there is another woman who has not had a successful procedure and eventually requires more surgery.

The red flag for any plastic surgeon performing this operation is the woman who has already had two or more operations and the breasts are still not symmetrical, soft, and pleasing to look at. Both the patient and the surgeon are frustrated, costs for each successive surgery are mounting, and she wants to know when the surgeon will get it right. At this point, many women who go on to become plaintiffs get at least one or more separate opinions on what went wrong. This is when the die is cast for also seeking out a plaintiff's attorney.

Why do women getting breast augmentation require two, three, or four and more secondary surgeries? Much of this can be explained by capsular contracture, scarring, and pocket problems. Studies suggest that contracture, scarring around the implant that can become painful, hardened, and misshape the breast, occurs in higher rates than has been published. After nearly 50 years of experience with implants of all kinds, surgeons still have not solved this riddle. The best solution to keeping this unfortunate circumstance from leading to a malpractice claim is still informed consent including a frank discussion with the patient before the surgery of who will be responsible for the fees for the surgery needed to remove the scar tissue formed around the implant. These are not inexpensive operations and the patient whose breasts respond with more scarring rather than less after secondary surgery will have a difficult time trying not to blame the surgeon for her problems.

While some of the secondary procedures in breast augmentation surgery can be explained by women changing their minds, wanting to have a bigger implant after all, or a scar that just simply needs a simple revision to look better, much of the revision surgery done after an augmentation is in fact to get a better mirror image from one side to the other. When that is successful and the patient has an admirable result with nothing to object to, the operation has become a success. But many of the re-operative surgeries in breast augmentation are not that simple.

Performing a full breast lift to tighten a loose skin envelope while also inserting an implant runs a very high risk of secondary surgery. Scars that become uneven and hypertrophic account for some of these complaints. But the more extreme problems are due to tension at the time of closure, leading to dehiscence, infections, and tissue necrosis and ultimately unsightly scarring that the patient was not prepared for no matter what she was told prior to surgery. Once again, these are the patients who have more than just one or two surgeries; many have gone on to two or more surgeons to seek a fix. Once healed, they are rarely ever happy that the surgery was done at all and will require a lot of attention emotionally from a caring surgeon to avoid seeking retribution.

In most of these cases, at some point there will have been a demand letter sent from the patient to the initial surgeon. Often long and filled with emotion, the letter will insist that the surgeon pay for all the costs associated with the next surgery, proposed by the plastic surgeon who has announced he or she is fully capable of rectifying all the problems, but at a cost often much higher than that of the original procedure. Each surgeon must make up his or her mind at this point what to do, but the first step should be to get personal help from the company who supplies his or her malpractice policy. In many instances, short of mediation, this is the last and best chance to try to keep the situation under control. Surgeons can make this work, avoiding a trip to the courthouse but usually not on their own. Signed disclaimers that the patient will agree not to sue in lieu of refunds can work but only when done correctly. Handling a demand letter should never be done by the surgeon alone.

Rhinoplasty

This operation when done right will often result in happy patients, but does it always mean these men and women will admit they have had their nose altered? In most instances, no. The nose is the only single non-paired organ that cannot be covered up from public viewing when operated on. And therein lies the key to claims for rhinoplasty. When something goes wrong in this operation, like in rhytidectomies, there is little the patient can do to hide the results from everyone who sees them.

Like breast augmentation, the key to unhappiness with this surgery is the failure after two or more operations to achieve a final outcome the patient can be satisfied with. But a less than satisfactory cosmetic outcome in many instances does not equate to negligence by itself. Something else usually affects the nose as well when the new shape alone did not make the patient happy.

Claims that go on to become problematic and involve more than just the cosmetic result more often involve a secondary side effect of the procedure, such as airway difficulty, a perforated septa and chronic rhinitis being among the main reasons. It is the annoying limited airway combined with even the most minor complaint about the appearance of the shape of the nose that makes the patient seek out an attorney. His or her unhappiness not only goes on unabated, but he or she is reminded of the problem with nearly every breath he or she takes, especially when they suffered no airway compromise before the surgery.

Patients who love the shape of their new nose can usually live with a compromised airway, and many do even as they admit that it is a problem. Patients whose nose annoys them in the mirror every time they look at themselves and whose unhappiness is magnified by airway complaints are the most common source of claimants for this procedure.

Liposuction

When this procedure is correctly performed, even the most satisfied patient can still have a minor irregularity in the skin, a ripple here, and a slight indentation there, that in certain lighting conditions or positions can be almost imperceptible. This is a side effect of the operation, no matter what type of liposuction instrument, technique or cannula was used. Patients who pursue claims against plastic surgeons after this procedure usually have much more problematic reasons to be unhappy.

The source of many of these complaints when claims data for this operation are studied is frankly poor patient selection. If the patient has poor skin tone to begin with, simply removing the underlying fat will not magically restore the outer skin envelope back to that of a teenager. When the end result is something that requires full clothing to cover up at the beach or eliminates the dip in the pool except alone, the average patient will not only be unhappy, but will also want retribution if they were promised something else completely.

Over-promising what liposuction can do is the primary source of patient complaints from this procedure. When it did not turn out right but the harm is little, the average attorney these days will tend to not take on this type of patient. When the disappointed patient however also has an uneven, asymmetrical result with ripples in the skin, significant depressions in areas where there should not be any, and painful nerve endings, the attorney will be much more likely to get an expert and then decide whether or not to file a claim.

Rarely, catastrophic results from suction lipectomy can and do occur. A perforated bowel, or a massive hematoma can occur regardless of the tools used and are considered to be results outside of the standard of care. Chronic pain from laser assisted devices that permanently affected nerve endings in the subcutaneous compartment is considered a side effect that can be defended but can also elicit tremendous sympathy from a jury as well.

In the end, most patients, when they are unhappy with the smoothness of their results from liposuction cannot these days expect to take a claim for their mild disappointment all the way to a courthouse. This in the end by itslef relegates this operation to a lower rank on the risk index scale than the volume of procedures alone might suggest.

Laceration repair

Taking emergency room calls for plastic surgery is either fraught with too much exposure to litiginous patients, or is a duty every surgeon owes to the hospital. The opionion varies significantly depending on which practitioner one speaks to. The bottom line is that this is usually a highly mobile population, they are often inebriated, and follow up can be essentially problematic to non-existent. Few patients who sustain significant trauma are ever happy with the scar no matter who repaired it. Claims in these situations have little to do with the time of the night the surgeon dropped what he or she was doing to respond to it and a lot more to do with retribution for the scar itself.

Two situations however bring many of these problems to an attorney's office other than just a very large scar (whether it was repaired well or not). Overlooked nerve injuries can and do occur. The window of opportunity to repair the facial nerve when it has been damaged is usually optimal when this secondary surgery is executed in the first 2-3 weeks after the injury. When the emergency room specialist performs a local block, then calls the plastic surgeon, the standard of care is to insist that the patient return for evaluation of the nerve within days after the skin was closed since the ability to determine why it was not working after the lidocaine injections was not possible.

In many of these claims, the patients failed to keep the critical follow-up appointment so that the nerve injury went un-assessed for months, dooming the eventual repair to something less than successful. Defending such a claim is entirely possible but it is essential that any and all attempts to contact this patient after their emergency room encounter are well documented in the chart. Juries in this instance have little sympathy for the claimant and side with the physician who tried unsuccessfully to track down the patient.

However, the plastic surgeon who never informed his or her staff of the need to get some type of follow up on this patient, never even started a chart from the night of the repair, and billed excessively for the services will not be seen in a positive light by many jurists.

The second situation is the failure to diagnose secondary injuries in the hand. When tendon lacerations or nerve injuries go undetected at the same time as the laceration the closure, there is once again a chance that the surgeon may not see the patient again in order to re-assess the injury and make the correct diagnosis. The plastic surgeon whose training includes hand surgery will be held to a higher standard of care in this instance than the emergency room physician who most likely missed the injury as well. These cases can be defended in court but are affected significantly when the patient makes a good case for how the resultant complications have significantly affected his or her life.

Hand surgery

While lower on the list of procedures that might end in an unhappy patient, hand surgery in general is not completely risk-free for the surgeon. Whether this is a major part of the plastic surgeon's individual practice or plays a minor role, it is not the volume that leads to the risk here but the operations.

Median nerve injuries during carpal tunnel releases, open or closed, are a frequent source of litigation. Closed instrumentation, while improving, does not always provide protection from the occasion when anatomical variants occur, such as the recurrent thenar branch exiting the transverse carpal ligament in the path of the knife, rather than the more radial side of the wrist. Unfortunately, discovering that this injury took place takes months of serial exams to determine that the lack of improvement from the simple release is not due to the patient seeking secondary gain and he or she really needs to have the nerve repaired.

Secondary releases are fraught with scar tissue embedded into the nerve, making delicate removal of the two tissues from each other tedious. As the two are not color-coded, the chances of injury to key nerve bundles are possible and do occur. When patients have had three or more surgeries on the painful, increasingly less useful hand and may be facing more, they have plenty of reason to ask an attorney if there has been malpractice. Unfortunately, in this type of surgery there always seems to be an expert somewhere who will say yes.

When 15% of all lawsuits stemming from the emergency room involve a single bone in the wrist, there must be a reason. Scaphoid injuries, notoriously hard to diagnose on the initial evaluation are another source of frequent litigation in the specialty. The standard of care is to always suspect it, then rule it out with serial testing as the missed diagnosis will be much more difficult to treat when it is made correctly weeks and even months later.

Besides the initial diagnosis problem with scaphoid fractures, when surgery is needed due to displacement or non-union, it is also notorious for incomplete resolution of the problem, especially when it is done primarily for pain relief. When two or three surgeons have tried to get a normal, functioning wrist and all failed, the patient will be left wanting to investigate whether or not he or she should get help from a plaintiff's attorney next rather than more surgery. Once again, experts will not be hard to find who will freely point a finger in all directions.

Other sources of claims in hand surgery include, as with lacerations in general, the emergency room patient who fails to follow up with the surgeon, removes the splint off his or her fractured finger, and then gets a stiff digit over the next few months, blaming the on-call plastic surgeon for his or her difficulties.

Lastly, other categories that lead to litigation will include failure to diagnose cancers masquerading as benign tumors in the hand and wrist, and failed re-attachment of digits–litigation that fits the old aphorism that "No good deed in medicine will go unpunished."

Blepharoplasty

As previously stated, the risk for litigation when performing a simultaneous facelift with blepharoplasty is significantly weighted to facial scarring, hematomas, and nerve injuries. Rarely is the eyelid surgery the reason for an angry patient.

But side effects and complications from this operation, while rare, are usually more than annoying to the patient when they persist for many months after the surgery. These include dryness of the eyes requiring near constant treatment, ectropion that is symptomatic and unsightly, and rarely, vision changes after surgery. Many of these patients will require specialty care, treatments that may include additional surgery and always more expense. When the plastic surgeon is at a loss to provide a cure, they will also soon find themselves facing tough questions from the patient, such as what went wrong. Explaining that to a jury might be the final step in a sad chain of events.

SUMMARY

Knowing which surgery in this specialty will expose the surgeon to a higher risk can be informative, especially as this type of information was never before available. How each surgeon uses this knowledge is unpredictable. Hopefully this can and will lead to personal algorithms for each member of the specialty who uses this information to prevent becoming another legal statistic (or victim, depending on one's point of view.) More analysis might be possible in the future as well, such as key studies of these data by region, gender, and verdict amounts. Making a science of these situations is possible, but fortunately in the end, the vast majority of plastic surgeons continue to do superb operations, make people happy with the results, and follow the standard of care in all of the situations they undertake.

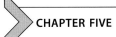

CHAPTER FIVE

The Unique Aspects of the Male Patient and Aesthetic Surgery

Are men different from women? Yes, of course they are and in so many ways. But the contrasts are not confined to just the obvious physical differences. There are also many emotional differences as well. Do the sexes vary when it comes to plastic surgery? Yes again. And the answer is that there are significant and important psychological disparities that come to bear when men and women pursue cosmetic surgery. From the initial consultation to the postoperative healing phase, the energy, reactivity, and situational adjustments can be exceedingly contradictory between the genders. The smart plastic surgeon knows this and adjusts his or her planning for the surgery accordingly.

What men say they want from any cosmetic surgery procedure can be totally opposite from that of a woman. Men also can be reticent to express why they are pursuing cosmetic surgery at all. Women pour their hearts out to anyone who will listen to their rationale. Yes, these differences can blur by personality type and are not always hard and fast. But plastic surgeons reading this will know exactly what this means. Gender differences in the exam room are very real.

Most women want their surgery to make them more attractive, as well as younger in appearance, often times fixing a nagging physical feature that has bothered them since youth.

Many men however will ask if the results from surgery will help them compete. They worry that younger workers might seem more eligible for that job opening everyone wants. Or they feel compelled to look more youthful so as to compete for women in a much younger age group. Interestingly, as society blurs the lines between the genders in regards to social power so can the rational for plastic surgery become reversed these days as well. Women living with men many years their junior will get tired of assumptions by strangers that it is a parental relationship and not a partnership. Comments such as "How nice to be taking your son out to dinner" drive them crazy. They want plastic surgery to reverse the hint that they are simply growing old.

On the other hand, traditionally when there is a difference of a decade or two between the man and the young woman dining together, the usual assumption that this is a romantic liaison can be and often is true. Those who inquire are surprised when the woman really is the progeny not the girlfriend. Society has tolerated the cradle-robbing divorced man for many years but it has taken a long time for it to adjust to the opposite gender, the older woman doing the same with much younger men. And for women, society has even given it a name, "cougar," when no such trendy moniker exists for the same behavior in men. This is the one area of cosmetic surgery where motivation merges between the sexes.

Men requesting facial cosmetic surgery are therefore increasingly just as determined to avoid "growing old gracefully" as women have been for the last century, although they express themselves quite differently. They do, however still resist skin treatments, mostly because they were never taught by their peers that it was an essential ingredient needed to stay "fresh" looking. Men with rugged good looks do not need applications of anything to the skin to stay that way. Skin care for men still has a long uphill battle to fight.

In the instance of the man seeking to stay younger to compete with the more youthful suitors, is it vanity or just another acquisition? Sociologists have a field day with this question, linking it to the harem behavior in herds of say, elk, deer, and sea lions. Men seeking to retain their youth to be attractive to the opposite sex will have a track record of many relationships, and are rarely married to their original partner when they request surgery. Men refuse to grow old gracefully for far different reasons than women.

Few men, if asked, will spend much time pondering this equation or even questioning it at all. More than women they see plastic surgery as a necessary (though possibly evil) tool towards meeting an end. And the end is finding youthfulness, in a partner and in the end themselves. Women are more likely to name wrinkles as the reason for facial surgery; men are more likely to talk about the loss of their youthful attractiveness. Women ask how to avoid looking worse. Men want to be sexier. Cosmetic surgery facilitates both of these desires. But the reasoning behind these choices will dictate how the surgeon deals with the patients, their anxieties, their motivation, and their potential for a smooth recovery before the surgery is even scheduled.

Over the past two decades there has been a steady increase in the number of men having cosmetic surgery, although it is still less than 10% of all procedures performed by members of American Society of Plastic Surgeons.

For men, rhinoplasty is the most often requested procedure followed by blepharoplasty, liposuction, gynecomastia reduction, and hair transplantation. Botox injections and laser hair removal are also popular male non-invasive procedures. Tummy tucks, while not unheard of in men, are not at the top of the list. Men can be just as embarrassed by how they look in clothes but they benefit from less beltline anxiety than their female counterparts. There is a well-known trend towards "mommy makeovers," fixing all that changed after pregnancy in one operation. There is no such corresponding surgery for dads outside of bariatric surgery, the removal of hanging loose skin after extreme weight loss.

Morphologically, there is a significant gender difference in the lower extremity and buttocks areas that affects the differential request for liposuction procedures between the sexes. Few men are affected by excess fat in the thighs or the buttocks. Lipodystrophy in men is carried in the trunk, including lower abdominal regions and the chest. Liposuction in the lower extremity is truly a female surgery.

Does the increase in men pursuing plastic surgery mean that they are all well suited for the challenges of recovering from a procedure? Possibly not. How men approach the surgery and tolerate the after affects can be so different than women that some plastic surgeons feel that few men are emotionally capable of making a smooth recovery. Men in general make more difficult patients than women. They complain more, fuss more over small items, and have lower tolerance of pain and complications. They can be extremely demanding of the surgeon both before and after the procedure to the point that both can end up regretting the entire undertaking. More than one wife has explained her husband's emotional roller coaster after surgery this way: "Men have never really had to endure a bad haircut. How could they possibly be prepared for looking temporarily horrible from surgery? They just are not wired for it."

Assuming these generalizations are true, is there then a way to determine which men will make good candidates for surgery and who might be better off just frankly turned down for their requests? To some extent yes. There are some important things for the surgeon to anticipate that should give guidance when making the right judgment call during the consultation with a male patient. While making the right decision may not always prevent a stressful situation from occurring, it might predict that this man will need some more attention in the perioperative period than a woman about to undergo the same surgery.

APPROPRIATE RATIONALE FOR SURGERY

Men who cannot verbalize easily why they want to change their appearance will need some extra time to determine if what they are requesting is actually reasonable. This is especially true if a spouse or significant other does the talking for them. The question arises then, who wants this more? In male facial cosmetic surgery, the danger is that the potential patient has no clue what his new appearance may or may not look like, but he is simply tired of the urging from the significant other to get something done. While reticence in itself will not indicate a poor candidate for surgery, a passive person may not be able to easily tolerate a complication, blaming everyone else for a poor result when they did not want to undertake the surgery in the first place anyway.

Emotionally inadequate men who are true power-seekers will also be unable to verbalize why they want to change their appearance. They might respond to anything that seems to challenge their inferiority complex with their own challenge, such as statements like, "What do you mean Doc, can't you not see why I am here?" Feelings of inadequacy in general can translate to unrealistic expectations from the surgery. Anxiety is normal when it comes to a professional consultation. Dealing with it through ridicule or inappropriate verbalization might be a red flag that trouble lies ahead.

These men when looking at themselves in the mirror after surgery are frequently confrontational, difficult to deal with, and fearful that they were exploited no matter how successful the surgeon considers the result. Their ability to handle any complication with grace and comfort will be nonexistent. They will demand answers when the problem has been explained already many times. Knowing when to turn this type of character down for surgery will make the surgeon's life a lot easier.

Both the surgeon and the patient can have a healthy and happy result when the patient's rationale for the request is reasonable for the anatomic problem he or she presents with. A reasonably well-adjusted man, no matter what his station in life, should be able to verbalize and discuss freely how he might want to look after surgery, although some coaxing may be needed. Motivation that conforms to the degree of the deformity is absolutely critical.

The ability to adequately assess motivation, and therefore, whether or not the male patient is a good candidate for the procedure is sometimes overshadowed however by issues particular to the type-A male, the "alpha dog". This fellow is used to getting his way. He fails to see his relationship with the physician as one of an equal, wants to negotiate the price early on, and does not appreciate taking directions, since he is used to giving them. He sees cosmetic surgery as a purchase, not a service. As he must win at everything, he will try to keep the upper hand throughout the process, beginning to end.

This type of patient can be very satisfied with the results of an operation but makes a terrible patient if complications occur. As he tended to brush aside any discussion of the risks before surgery, he is surprised when he does not heal instantly overnight. Often this type has a passive spouse, one who finds it difficult to reinforce the need to follow directions, much less getting him to read them in the first place. He will often use his employed staff as a liaison to communicate with the office and the physician. He expects to have special attention at all times. These men will become well known to the surgeon's entire staff in no time, and not necessarily for good reasons.

FIXATION ON A FEATURE

Another red flag that can come to the forefront during the initial consultation with the plastic surgeon is a male patient who obsesses over one particular feature and clearly has a "hang up" with it. The acronym "SIMON" was coined many years ago and is still in common usage today by plastic surgeons to identify this unique type of male patient.

S-I-M-O-N stands for "Single, Immature, Male, Obsessed, and Narcissistic." These men are most likely to express extreme disappointment with the postoperative result than any other plastic surgery patient type. No amount of reassurance or encouragement during the healing phase can reduce their anxiety that things did not work out at surgery. They exhibit unreasonable amounts of apprehension and distress and can require near daily attention. Eventually, they can be satisfied but more often than not they only arrive at satisfaction after exhausting the surgeon and his or her staff.

Can one determine this obsessive behavior at the first consultation? Clues to this type of individual exist. Any male patient who has evidence of immature relationships with others, blames everyone else, especially his family, for his predicament in life, and exhibits overly secretive behavior such as insisting no one can know that he is even considering surgery, can be considered to have elements of this type of personality.

Evidence that this might be a person on whom not to operate can include complete failure to establish any rapport with the patient as well as significant indecisiveness, unending demands that perfection will be achieved, and the need for reassurance that the new appearance can be guaranteed.

Often, the history obtained from these individuals can include multiple other surgeries, multiple hospitalizations under unusual circumstances, and a medication history compatible with adjustment problems, depression, and anxiety disorders. They also can heap praise on the surgeon who will "save" them. They will site research to prove that they have chosen the right surgeon but simultaneously exhibit impulsiveness as well.

These individuals require a second or third consultation not only to determine that they indeed are good candidates for the surgery but also to determine that their support network is adequate. Anyone who insists on going to great lengths to secure privacy after surgery including enlisting the surgeon and staff in a ruse about the true nature of the operation is probably not going to be a satisfied patient. In the end, when the new feature looks significantly and obviously the result of surgery, he will be forced into denial and guess who will take the blame for that?

Many times these men will also be very specific about the postoperative appearance. Small details will seem overly important. They may stare at themselves incessantly during the consultation, to the point of distraction and with an inability to concentrate on what the surgeon is saying. They may bring photographs of others they wish to look like. Rarely do they bring anyone from a support network along with them, such as family and friends. This is especially true when they demand that the surgery must remain a total secret to others.

Dismissing these individuals can require diplomacy. Suggesting that they are overly obsessed with appearances and should not have surgery can be met with great objection and pleading. Alternately, suggesting therapy rather than surgery may not be met with consideration and agreement. The most appropriate way to disengage from these individuals without doing them a disservice is to be frank and open about what was revealed in the consultation. Admitting forthrightly to one's concerns that the patient is fixated and should concentrate on other qualities of their appearance may not be met with enthusiasm but is still the correct thing to do. When all else fails, suggesting a second and third opinion may allow the patient to hear the same conclusion often enough that it will eventually sink in.

MALE BREAST REDUCTION: A REQUEST THAT'S DIFFERENT

This is a unique request in plastic surgery, one where the direct physiological consequences of puberty, medications, or obesity can clash with self-image resulting in distress and embarrassment in otherwise well-adjusted young and even older men. Regardless of the reason for the enlargement (and facing the fact that in the majority of men it is idiopathic), providing a solution to the enlargement that restores the normal male physique can be rewarding. These men can be just as excited about their new chest as women undergoing breast enlargement.

The most reasonable request for male breast reduction comes from males who have tried to reduce their chest through diet and exercise only to be frustrated that this made little or no difference in the end. They are often healthy and have relationships that are effective for them in their daily lives. They are tired of covering up their chest in two or more layers of clothing and disappointed that they are self-restricted from the beach, the pool, or sports. They also make very grateful patients when clothing and social encounters need no longer to be calculated carefully.

However, there will also need to be a frank discussion about what the realistic results will be. Virtually all will have a breast glandular component as well as lipodystrophy contributing to the enlargement. Some will also have skin hypertrophy, to the point that the surgery will result in some skin scars, possibly quite extensive. In the end, a chest with multiple scars in several directions is just as likely to be covered up as the original problem was.

As with other men mentioned in this chapter, the degree of deformity is the clue to the likelihood of satisfaction after the surgery. Minimal breast enlargement without asymmetry can suggest obsessive behavior in the candidate. The desire to avoid any scars can be a clue as well that this might not be the best surgical candidate. Any patient who demands reassurances that they will look absolutely normal afterwards is someone who might best be turned down for the procedure. Demanding the problem be fixed only with liposuction is also a red flag as leaving glandular tissue behind can exacerbate the protruding nipple areolar complex and lead to equal concerns in clothing all over again.

VISCERAL LIPODYSTROPHY

Men requesting changes to their waistline must be carefully evaluated to avoid feeling cheated by abdominal liposuction. While many will have some degree of excess fat below the skin compartment, some will not. Middle aged men with a protruding abdomen that hangs over the belt line and gives them a barrel shape most often have hypertrophy of the fat lining the intestinal mesentery. Their abdominal musculature usually lies just below the thin subcutaneous compartment and juts outward from the ribs to the umbilicus, then swings sharply back to the pelvis. Their only hope of changing this is through diet and exercise. Suctioning off some fat will not bring about much change, but will certainly bring on a feeling they were over-sold on what the procedure would do. Rarely are they happy that their money was well spent.

Some of these morphologically distinct men also have lipodsytrophy, mostly at the side of the hips and the posterior trunk at the upper buttocks/lumbar region. While liposuction will definitely help in this limited area, patients must clearly be told where it will not make a difference.

Abdominoplasty on this type of abdomen before weight loss is also a poor choice and can lead to a disappointing outcome. Trying to plicate the abdominal musculature over a visceral compartment that is already protruding with its contents packed tightly into this space can lead to delayed healing of the incision, skin necrosis, pain, and a result that neither the surgeon nor the patient will be very proud of. Understanding this concept is key to avoiding a disastrous ending, and possibly a date in court. When the plastic surgeon misses these key physical signs, and operates anyway, the plaintiff's team will have little trouble finding an expert who can explain to the jury why the surgery never should have been done in the first place.

Knowing which men to turn down for this surgery is just as important as knowing how to do it on the right candidates.

CLAIMS FILED BY MEN

While fewer liability claims may be filed by men, it is most likely the result of fewer numbers of plastic surgery procedures being performed on them in general. When they do file, it is usually for the same reasons as that of a woman. Rhinoplasty procedures where breathing problems became worsened after the nose was reshaped are the focus in this most popular male operation. In blepharoplasty, constant eye dryness after an aggressive procedure with corneal exposure can drive both men and women eventually to a plaintiff's attorney.

Uneven and lumpy results in liposuction, obvious scars around the ears after a facelift, and the loss of hair and sensation from a browlift are the same problematic sources of anger in both sexes.

What has never been studied is whether men are more prone to seek compensation for their troubles than women. If this is due to the male tendency to spar over the consequences that seem unfair to them, it has not yet been formally realized. The other ripe area for study is whether men, angry over the result but embarrassed to admit they had surgery, are less likely to want to face a jury than a woman in a similar circumstance.

SUMMARY

Men increasingly are asking for the help of plastic surgeons. They are troubled by large noses, baggy eyelids, diet- and exercise-resistant fat along the belt line, feminized breasts, and wrinkled necks and jowls. When they are appropriately evaluated, taught carefully what to expect from the surgery, and have a successful outcome, they can be very happy patients and even occasionally refer additional patients to their surgeon. But the pitfalls in treating men must be understood. They require a very different approach than that of treating women and the entire office staff must be aware of this. When they have a bad outcome it becomes a source of tension. They can challenge the surgeon over things female patients accept readily. Men want instant recovery and can require an abundance of patience from the caregivers while they adjust to what has been done. The wise plastic surgeon understands all of this and plans for it accordingly.

CHAPTER SIX

Avoiding Liability in Reconstructive Surgery

While cosmetic surgery lawsuits seem to get all the attention, there are other areas of plastic surgery where liability problems exist as well. They may be less noticed, are often less conspicuous (even within the medical community), and the cases brought to trial are certainly fewer in number. But there can still be sensational details involved and juries in these trials will pay just as much attention to what transpired as if it was a cosmetic procedure they were likely to have seen on reality TV.

Cosmetic surgery can be defined as taking a normal structure and enhancing its appearance. Reconstruction therefore is defined as taking an abnormal structure and making it more normal. While there are a few "cross over" or gray areas such as rhinoplasty where the definitions can get somewhat blurred, this simple distinction between the two areas of plastic surgery cleanly segregates these theaters in most cases.

Certain types of reconstructive cases are the most frequently performed procedures in the specialty. These include "tumor" removal of all sorts, whether superficial or deep, and reconstructing the newly created defect with a closure designed to give a tidy result. This is still the mainstay operation of plastic surgeons and with the number of new skin cancers continuing to rise, it is unlikely this will change any time soon. While claims from these surgeries are less frequent than from other types of cancer-related surgery, when they occur, they usually are due to several unique pitfalls that occur most commonly.

Breast reconstruction, one of the areas where claims are filed in a very high proportion of cases, has already been discussed in Chapter 4. Hand surgery as well was discussed in that chapter and likewise ranks in the top 10 categories for all claims filed in this specialty. Two other types of reconstruction tend to make up the bulk of claims filed for non-cosmetic surgery. These are facial trauma and limb salvage. While both have their own unique problems that can trap the unfortunate surgeon, when a claim gets filed against the reconstructive surgeon, it is usually because of a limited number of reasons, no matter what the actual complications or end results may have been.

The bulk of these lawsuits are filed for claims of lack of informed consent and violations of the standard of care, with infection and unnecessary scarring often rounding out the list and frequently lumped in by the plaintiff's attorney for good measure. While each case will have its own particular merits, in general, all of the claims in this area of the specialty tend to fall into these few categories.

What is unique to many of the claims in reconstructive plastic surgery however is the concept of what constitutes "normal" appearance. When the patient expects to go back to his or her former lifestyle with his or her general appearance intact, their hopes can be dashed by surgery that was, however, successful by the surgeon's standards but in reality going out in public will have significant implications for them. Nearly normal still is not the same as absolutely normal. Covering up what used to be displayed openly, avoiding intimacy, and the eventual development of acute depression from ongoing loss of self-esteem, all tend to transpire in the end. The surgeon may feel he or she did their best. The patient however only sees the scars and is not happy with them.

In part, avoiding liability in reconstruction involves also managing patient expectations. In the days of huge headlines touting miracle cures, and constant television exposure to the details of celebrity cosmetic surgery, all too often the downfall of what the surgeon thinks is a successful reconstruction is the patient's assumption that miracles happen everyday and they are owed the semblance of a normal appearance. Patients can feel, "If it can be done for some why can't it be done for me?"

The surgeon's presumptions about restoration become irrelevant to a patient who is relatively media-crazed and expects not just restoration but a new perfect body because he or she has now had "plastic surgery." This attitude can prevail in discussions with the family as well, both before and after surgery. Whether the end result will be seen by a plaintiff's attorney as having merit depends on what the chart will reveal to him or her.

Relentless patients with little basis for a claim other than their disappointment with the result, used to be successful bringing their complaint to multiple attorneys until one agreed to take on the claim. But with the costs of bringing a case to trial increasing dramatically, many attorneys may now think twice about filing a claim when all they intended was a quick settlement and not a trial. The best defence strategy in these instances when there is little merit to a claim may be to offer nothing and eventually see the claim disappear altogether.

INFORMED CONSENT

It has been said that claims stemming from a perceived lack of informed consent are very winnable for the defense. When this is the only basis for the claim, this axiom may be mostly true.

While this is rarely the most important portion of the plaintiff's case, in most reconstructive cases the charge of lack of informed consent is thrown in routinely along with the kitchen sink to compound the charges of negligence. Rather than dismissing it as an irrelevant issue, the defense team must still deal with it separately at mediation, settlement, or trial. Whether or not an informed consent document will prevail in these instances depends on many factors. But having a poorly worded one or one that fails to go into detail at all about the planned reconstructive surgery digs a fairly big hole for the team to have to crawl out of at the start of a claim.

Yet this is precisely what happens in many situations where the surgery was performed in a teaching hospital and there is little accompanying documentation verifying what the patient was told. Often the patient undergoes a reconstructive procedure during an admission for trauma, possibly weeks after the original injury. In many cases the plastic surgery procedure was not the first or second surgery that took place during that admission. When the chart is reviewed by the plaintiff's counsel, one of the first things he or she will look for, and find often enough, is no dictation or chart note from an attending physician that a thorough discussion took place, explaining the risks to the patient in detail prior to a major reconstructive operation. The signed consent is a generic form provided by the hospital with usually no detail but lots of vague and general disclaimers. Juries can be easily convinced that this was not adequately applicable to the real details of a major plastic surgery case. When the patient was on continual narcotic medication prior to the surgery, it will be argued that he or she could not possibly have understood what was being presented to him or her anyway. The best way to avoid this scenario is to always have family members as witnesses to the consent process.

When side effects and complications occur after the surgery for whatever reason, the resulting anguish and prolonged additional recovery might have been avoidable, but certainly the risk for this should have also been anticipated. Regardless of what the reason for the surgical failure, if the patient suffers the loss of additional tissue, or has significant side effects and complications prolonging his or her hospital stay, the first part of the defense of this claim will hinge in part on the jury's assessment of what the patient really understood before he or she agreed to the surgery. Were they told everything they needed to know to have made a clear decision to proceed, knowing what the chances of a poor outcome were? Too often, even if this discussion took place, there is no evidence to show a jury that the decision was made after a full and clear risk assessment took place at the bedside with or without the family.

Residents in teaching hospitals have their hands full as it is. Getting the surgery schedule right and the patient prepped for the case takes priority. Delegating the consent to the most junior member of the team happens all the time. But at this point in their careers, few of these young men and women have the experience to explain all the risks and alternatives in detail, especially if they are rotating through the service from their own specialty training and know little about reconstruction.

Attending surgeons should give long and hard thought to carrying out this responsibility. When they do, it is also imperative that they take the time to get what transpired during their time with the patient in writing, in prompt fashion. When informed consent is properly carried out, the rare case that then goes on to a full-blown claim will find both the malpractice insurance provider and the defense attorneys armed with the right tools for a successful defense of the informed consent portion of the claim.

ALTERNATIVE PROCEDURES

When patients whose reconstruction went poorly suffer from prolonged recovery, including multiple corrective surgeries or even an amputation, they will always wish it had gone quicker and smoother. When they find out that an alternative surgery existed and they were not made aware of it, it is only natural for them to assume that they missed a chance to have a totally different outcome. When the claim gets filed in these instances, this is exactly what the plaintiff's expert will tell the jury. The emphasis will be on the failure to give the patients all the facts they needed to have made a different, perhaps smarter, decision. It is not hard to find experts willing not only to testify to this but also to point out that they always use the alternative approach themselves and have zero complications from it. What is the jury to do? They will side with the most credible expert, the one they could relate to most on an emotional level, regardless of whose side they were on.

This scenario happens all too often in breast reconstruction as was pointed out in Chapter 4. If a muscle-based flap failed and the patient was left with significant additional scars, they will claim they should have been offerred a tissue expander and an implant. The same holds true for patients who get an immediate reconstruction with an implant. After multiple surgeries trying to get the breast to look like something more than a glob on the chest, and after multiple attempts to get rid of capsular contracture, they will meet sooner or later another patient who had the alternative surgery, a muscle based flap, which went smoothly. The assumption is that had they known "the truth" about every alternative, they never would have picked the one that went so wrong.

This also holds true for limb salvage procedures and complex wrist surgery. If there truly are two or three other ways to perform the reconstruction, each and every one must be spelled out, including why the one that is preferred by the surgeon is being chosen in this instance. Patients do not retain much of these discussions. But not discussing the alternatives at all gives them nothing to retain, and every reason to suspect that they got railroaded into the surgeon's favorite type of procedure once they learn there was some other way to do it. Since patients' memories can get exhausted in a long hospitalization, it is imperative to document in the chart that these alternatives were offered as well.

VIOLATIONS OF THE STANDARD OF CARE

What constitutes the standard of care in reconstruction can often be contentious. At deposition and trial, the experts will not be hard to find for each side of the argument. Some of what took place during the hospitalization and recovery in reconstruction may not be confined to plastic surgery standards but are really general standards for all surgery. Wound care, antibiotic therapy, and outpatient follow-up care are the same no matter what the specialty. Treating patients with diabetes, hypertension, and congestive heart failure differs very little from specialty to specialty.

The contention that plastic surgeons performing reconstruction were not qualified to also do the general postoperative care should carry little weight at trial. On the basis of a long history of training in general surgery, the specialty includes adequate learning skills to deal with many situations. But in the instance where a missed diagnosis of a true non–surgical complication transpired and a consultant was not brought in, the defense problems will be multiplied.

Applying the same standard of care for all surgeons to a plastic surgeon performing reconstruction will be difficult for some juries to grasp. The skills of the defense team can be critical to get a layperson to profess that a consultant was unnecessary. When the ward treatment of a complication failed however, there will be no shortage of specialists who will freely testify that it could have been avoided if the consultant came in on time. This issue alone may not be the one that runs a case, but in conjunction with other issues at a trial, it may paint a picture of less than stellar postop care, or to a plaintiff's attorney, plain old incompetence. Knowing the standard of care in treating patients with pre-existing secondary diagnoses will avoid this situation. Failing that, the best care is to simply call for help early and often.

INFECTIONS

No one ever plans to allow a postop infection. To a surgeon, it is a side effect, avoidable through the judicious use of perioperative antibiotics. To a plaintiff's attorney, however, an infection that led to other severe issues is always seen as a complication. The jury will get a withering string of experts testifying that the infection was avoidable, that the wrong antibiotics were used, and that other means should have been used to avoid the offending bacteria. These issues can all be argued in front of a jury with sound medical basis and facts.

Less easy to defend, however, is the abject failure to recognize an infection at all. Patients discharged with swollen extremities and low grade fevers who then become septic at home within a day of discharge will get a thorough review from an interested attorney. When the infection leads to the loss of a reasonable result from the reconstructive surgery, finger pointing will begin. A surgical abscess that went unrecognized will surely be painted as a mistake, regardless of how subtle the presenting signs were. When this prolongs the patient's recovery for months and racks up six figures in hospital costs, the jury will be asked to answer who should be the ultimate source of blame. This is the scenario in some cases where even the most adroit physicians would not have been able to predict the impending disaster without so much as a hint of physical signs. But if important lab tests were misinterpreted, or worse, never seen until it was too late, the focus of a plaintiff's case will be to paint an inglorious picture of a surgeon out of touch and providing inappropriate care.

How does the plastic surgeon avoid becoming ensnared in this scenario? Some rely heavily on prophylaxis; others feel this choice only delays the inevitable and contributes to the widespread problem of bacterial resistance. Whichever side the embattled surgeon decided to choose, the plaintiff's side will find an expert to rebut that stance after a vicious infection wrecked havoc with the reconstruction. Doing the right thing can be interpreted in many ways. Defending whichever choice was made will unfortunately depend heavily on which side's expert is able to persuade the jury best.

Once again, the best defense for a surgical infection lies with an informed consent process, one that clearly spelled out that infections are always possible and the results from them can mean loss of life or limb. Will it scare patients unnecessarily? It possibly will do so; but on the other hand, it also sends a strong message that the surgical team is looking ahead to every eventuality. Many patients by now have heard something about hospital-borne infections. Many may know someone suffered from one. Denying them any information at all preoperatively will look like a surgeon's poor behavior pattern of denial and lack of openness to a jury, which they may not take keenly to.

SCARRING

To many reconstructive surgeons faced with a large open wound, the issue of getting it closed in one stage takes precedence over the issue of a cosmetically challenging donor site scar. It is more likely that a bedside discussion will focus on which flap is the appropriate choice for what needs to be covered when both surgeon and patient are anxious about the hole staring them both in the face. It also however should always include the effects on the donor site, both functional and cosmetic. There will be pros and cons for each flap chosen by the surgical team. Each open wound will dictate its own need for muscle or other tissue, not just skin and dermis. Getting too wrapped up in the choice of flaps will often lead the surgeon to ignore the fact that there are always considerations to be made about the patient's acceptance of a large donor site scar, no matter how heroic the closure was.

When a surgeon tells the patient nothing about this donor scar in advance, does it condemn the defense of a claim filed much later for just that reason? Not necessarily. A good defense team can explain to a jury that the end result, a salvage of a terrible situation, could not have occurred without the required donor tissue. But when this scar is included in the full pre-operative discussion, the resultant appearance will have little basis as the only reason to file a claim against the surgeon; especially when it is documented that the patient knew what the result would be.

In reality, the scarring that leads a patient to file a claim is just one of a number of reasons he or she is unhappy. But a long heavy scar in itself can become the nagging reminder he or she sees everyday, the evidence that something must have gone wrong, something he or she wasn't told about, the fodder that stirs up the desire for restitution. Having to explain it to curious friends and strangers gets old over time. Donor site scars often limit the type of clothing one can wear. In the case of some patients, eventually they simply give up and live with the fact that exposing it will lead to stares and comments. Only a few patients learn how to avoid being frustrated by this.

The radial forearm flap is a classic example of a donor site that is cosmetically difficult to hide. The trade off for this donor site must be explained in detail, then the discussion documented in the chart, including what was said about future correction of the donor site. This is absolutely necessary to defer later disappointment and retribution when patients claim they would not have allowed this surgery had they known what it would mean to them permanently later on. It is a terrific flap in the right circumstance. It is also a terrifically problematic donor site. A surgeon who uses it regularly can get lax when describing the resulting defect to a patient in need of it. Leaving out important details such as this can surely come back to haunt the hurried and the harried surgeon.

Finally, the surgeon must anticipate the patient's inherent tendency to form poor scars based on their skin type and color as well as inherited factors, and discuss fully what might result. Patients can accept large scars when they know it was the only alternative. Returning to a full active lifestyle because of reconstructive surgery means trade offs. Juries will understand that there may have been little alternative. When the surgeon documented that this was spelled out in advance, the defense will become strengthened. The more desperate the need was for this tissue and the better the discussion was about the alternatives, the less chance there will be that a jury will be sympathetic to the plaintiff's complaints about a large scar. But if other issues such as an infection prevail in court *and* the patient displays a horrific donor scar he or she wasn't told about, juries may have trouble rooting for the surgeon.

FACIAL TRAUMA

The repair of facial fractures that ultimately finds the surgeon defending themselves in court can be classified into two types: those that require dental alignment and everything else that doesn't. Non-unions and malunions of the maxilla and the mandible constitute much of the bulk of claims from facial trauma. With multiple approaches to fixation, the two sides in court will both be able to make persuasive arguments as to the reason that the one used was either right or wrong. The defense will often point to the patient's poor postoperative participation or lack thereof as the source of the problem. The extent of the original injury will also be an issue when the bite is malaligned permanently. This type of contentious case will also include inter-specialty comparison of techniques as the repair of these fractures is shared among three or more specialties.

As in other areas of reconstructive surgery, the possibility of corrective surgery must be spelled out to the patient early on. The costs of the secondary surgery frequently are the catalyst for unhappiness. Secondary problems at the TMJ joint which may have pre-dated the trauma can also trigger a lawsuit when pain intervenes at every meal after an emergency operation, but may have been inevitable any way. Was the trauma patient informed of this eventuality? Often he or she was told very little about the long-term consequences, and are the ones that will bring the case to the courthouse in the first instance.

The preparation for taking a facial trauma patient to surgery for major realignment and fixation should always include a thorough discussion of the potential for permanent loss of function to all the vital structures that will be encountered. This should include the potential for the loss of sensory nerve functions, changes in vision including the possibility of permanent loss of sight, as well as loss of smell, taste, and the other senses. The potential for the loss of facial animation due to damage to the facial nerve should be laid out before surgery is undertaken.

Documenting what facial functions worked and didn't work before the reconstruction took place is as important to the eventual defense of a claim as choosing the correct fixation techniques. Failing to document this prior to surgery will mean that a lot more work will have to be done in the defense of an eventual claim than if it had been clearly laid out in the chart in the first place. A plaintiff's attorney perusing a chart before making a decision to file a claim can be easily dissuaded from going forward when it is obvious that the surgical team took a thorough stance to protect themselves for just that eventuality.

LIMB SALVAGE

Expectations are everything in this category. With exposed hardware at the fracture site, impending osteomyelitis and a poor prognosis that the limb can be salvaged, the plastic surgeon who steps in to cover the wound will be expected by everyone to be a hero and save the day. They may also have that attitude. Regardless of these expectations, it is imperative to approach the problematic wound with the goals for surgery clearly explained directly in front of the patient. There will be scars from a donor site, and if muscle is being harvested the potential for a deficit of strength from the loss of that tissue should be spelled out as well. The potential failure rate of free flaps should be dicussed, as well as what will occur if the vascularization of the limb fails. Alternatives for bone and hardware coverage may become out of the question at that point and the next steps should be discussed frankly. When this is also adequately documented in the chart, there is a basis for defense that most juries will understand.

Too often what is missed at this point is a blunt and candid discussion of the recovery phase, such as how long it might take before normal ambulation will, if ever, be accomplished. More importantly, the alternative, such as the time it might take to walk more normally with an immediate amputation and a prosthetic fitted within a month must also be discussed, especially when this might lead to shorter hospitalization. As with all reconstructions, the alternative operation, in hindsight, will always look better to a patient who has had to struggle to regain function and claims he or she wasn't given all the facts to make the right decision.

The team that tells the patient everything will be normal after limb salvage surgery sets themselves up for a difficult defense when in reality what is normal after limb salvage may be anything but that. Yes, there will be a foot, and yes, the leg may be somewhat normal in appearance. While the success rate in this surgery is remarkable and many patients are grateful for having their leg saved and going on to live a near normal life, some patients will also find themselves in financial debt and stress after the trauma. The attitude that "the doctors who left me looking like a freak should pay" is often just what some plaintiff attorneys find irresistible. Add to this a sloppy hospital chart with multiple missing documents and a poorly carried out informed consent process, and you have the makings for a hotly contested lawsuit. Why would anyone make it easy for a patient to pursue this course of action?

TUMOR REMOVAL

The issues here are not that much different from those of the other areas of reconstruction. Adequate removal of the tumor with clear margins, lymph node dissection when needed, and closure of the defect in a tidy fashion leave little room for complaint. What does it take to make a case for the jury when it seems that all of this was done appropriately? Mostly it is driven by recurrence or spread of the tumor, flaps that were too bulky but never were re-operated, and failure to inform the patient of the reality of his or her appearance after all is said and done.

As previously noted this is a very frequent procedure in plastic surgery. The pitfalls for even the most experienced surgeon however usually include consequences that were completely within his or her control and should have been anticipated. Incomplete removal with subsequent recurrence of a tumor that was thought to be eradicated once and for all *can* happen. Is this negligence? Many a plaintiff's attorney has concluded it is, and he or she has then aggressively pursued the position that an alternative method (that the surgeon didn't choose) for checking margins and getting a final clear pathology report was the only possible course of action.

Patients also do not take kindly to learning after the fact that there may have been alternatives to a disfiguring surgery. With the debate about Moh's chemosurgery becoming the standard of care as an alternative to frozen section margin control, there will always be an expert waiting in the wings to testify that the plastic surgeon should have offered this as an alternative. In many instances, such as eyelid and nasal tumors as well as some recurrences, it is indeed becoming a reliable and often- used technique. But it is not 100% foolproof, which must be pointed out to a jury when this becomes the pivotal issue in a tumor recurrence claim.

If Moh's chemosurgery was not considered, the plaintiff's attorney will have no trouble finding an expert to claim its advantages. If it was offered to the patient but not documented in the chart, it might as well not have been discussed. If the recurrence resulted in disfigurement, as can occur with even non-aggressive basal or squamous cell skin cancers, the surgeon does himself a great favor to point out this possibility before he or she performs the original surgery and not afterward.

In some of these cases, the surgeon did not have a system for thoroughly reviewing the pathology report, so that clues to an incomplete removal were ignored. This then can go on to become the turning point of a malpractice case when the patient later suffers a recurrence of the cancer along with all of the consequences, and the chart becomes a smoking gun. It is imperative that every pathology report be verified, signed, and dated by the surgeon as a protection to avoid this phenomenon. Letting just one aberrant report slip through the cracks can lead to a long protracted claim that will cause extended regrets on everyone's part.

The informed consent issue must always include a discussion about the possibility of incomplete removal, how it would be dealt with, and recurrence of the tumor. If the patient chooses to go somewhere else after hearing a frank discussion about this the surgeon may be better off for the effort. Failing to discuss these scenarios before the surgery or failing to document that it took place will leave a busy tumor surgeon exposed at some point to the question.

With any tumor removal then the wise surgeon protects himself or herself with a discussion about these issues beforehand and includes the facts that were discussed in a chart note proving that this took place. Offering the alternative approaches, spelling out the possibility of recurrence, tissue damage, or incomplete tumor removal, and signing off on the pathology report with the date it was reviewed will show any jury that the surgeon was aware of these issues. When he or she can prove that he or she made the patient aware of them as well, any claims to the contrary usually disappear.

In summary then, reconstruction in plastic surgery is not without the possibility of errors. How this is safeguarded by the surgeon and the staff, how the informed consent is carried out, and how infections and complications are dealt with do not guarantee a happy patient. But they will ensure that the defense of any claims from an litiginous patient will have adequate grounds to protect the surgeon in this eventuality.

CHAPTER SEVEN

The Psychological Aspects of Modifying a Patient's Anatomy

There are a myriad of factors that constitute the psychology of changing one's appearance. Internal motivation, external motivation from relationships with the opposite sex, skeletons in the closet left from one's parents and siblings, obsession with a feature not that abnormal in its appearance, all these things are terribly important to assess for a surgeon trying to decide on whom to perform elective surgery. Yet unfortunately nothing about this subject is at all a part of the curriculum of training for a young cosmetic surgeon. These important factors are left to become part of the "on-the-job" training; while some learn from their mistakes, other surgeons seem doomed to repeating them. Despite the lengthy training a surgeon goes through, many fail to acquire the basic criteria for determining appropriate patient selection. Most learn from experience later in life and basically from a long history of seeking to understand what makes up a patient with the right, not the wrong, motivation. Unfortunately, some never ask that question.

Pool a group of plastic surgeons who have been in practice for less than 5 years and one most likely would get a general agreement that there are patient types that they would prefer never to operate on again. Despite having been trained in the latest techniques in the specialty, none of them will recall being schooled in the important arena of patient selection. It seems there is no longer enough time to learn all the skill sets in the specialty as it is, let alone the gray areas. What they now know about the subject was learned through trial and error once they started to practice. This has been the same paradigm for the specialty since its inception 80 plus years ago.

This is unfortunate for those who deal with the liability issues of this specialty, as much of what turns a procedure into malpractice is based on the psychological interaction between the surgeon and the patient.

This problem is confounded by the increasing love affair between the media and plastic surgery, both the good results and the less than successful ones. The Hollywood media, in particular, has built unreal expectations for success in one's vocations based on plastic surgical changes to one's anatomy. The tempo of this hype is inescapable. The simple act of buying groceries forces one to wait in a line facing the front pages of the tabloid media, most of which place the latest results of surgery on the rich and famous on the cover with blaring headlines declaring if it was good, bad, or ugly. Television is no less guilty.

Normal patients have normal filters. The act of deciphering for oneself what the message is from all this and adding one's own reality check to it is a normal filter. Being able to understand that the media makes a frenzy out of everything and then discarding as fantasy most of what is passed by one's eyes and ears is what makes up being normal. One should decide for one's own self what is the message, what is reality, and what is just for fun. Truly well-adjusted individuals will add their own interpretation, and this is part of being well balanced. Patients who instead internalize the media message for themselves and then cannot accept their own physical appearance without these filters on the message may not make good patients and may have difficulty accepting any result after surgery.

So what about the patient whose filters are not mature, who are susceptible to these messages, who have internalized the message that you will not be accepted in society with abnormal appearances? Label these types as immature or unrealistic; it is highly important that they be evaluated correctly before the surgeon agrees to operate on them. Can they become happy patients after cosmetic surgery? Some do but only when properly prepared for the traumatizing aspects of recovery, and when their expectations of what the result will do for them have been tailored by the surgeon. They do not do well when they enroll for surgery in a busy "puppy mill," a practice where nonskilled assistants do the work of signing up the patient and the surgeon fills the role of just another technician, hardly knowing the patient at all before the surgery.

Those who perform cosmetic surgery must also have filters, but of a much different type. To always do the right operation on the right patient means filtering out those whose motivation is perhaps inappropriate. One must also filter out those who will have the ability to withstand a less than perfect result while awaiting a second surgery to correct it. And filtering out the patient whose support system is totally based on others' opinions, not his or her own, is a critical skill that takes years of experience. Even surgeons who have been at this for years will occasionally have to admit they got it wrong and that they missed a key warning sign before surgery took place.

However, failing to ever look into the motivation of any patient can doom the results for both surgeon and patient, no matter how perfectly the surgery was performed. Eventually, the wrong patient will get the wrong procedure and there will be hell to pay. This is the genesis of many a malpractice case in this specialty.

THE INTERFACE BETWEEN SURGEON AND PATIENT MOTIVATION

Short of being born with a sixth sense for determining what makes a good plastic surgery patient and which patients should be turned away, there are some working paradigms that can help this situation. Much of it involves asking a few key questions of each new patient, then pursuing the answers with follow-up questions.

Asking the open-ended question involves some commitment on the part of the surgeon. It is far different than the questioning involved in taking a medical history. The skills needed to interpret the answers, however, can be learned relatively quickly. Steering the conversation back to motivation regardless of how chatty the patient gets is a skill set that needs some practice. An endless string of thoughts away from the subject can indicate a patient unable to recognize the reasoning for this intake discussion and will require patience to get things back on track.

By no means do the following questions come from a psychologically tested and verified instrument. In fact, they are simply the ways in which the authors have found down through the past half century that they can drill down quickly into the patient's motivations and, with a reasonable level of reassurance, prove for themselves that they have a patient who is correctly motivated for surgery and can withstand the onslaught of problems that might take place in the recovery period.

1. "If you could wave a magic wand and change anything about yourself, what would you do?"
2. "What will this procedure do for you when it is all over?"
3. "Do you know anyone else who has had plastic surgery, and were they happy about it?"
4. "What will people who know you think about you when they find out about this?"
5. "I see you are married; who wants this procedure more, you or your spouse?"

Answers to these questions and others like them should be straightforward. A person whose motivations are authentic and original will be able to respond easily to these questions and describe his or her wants deliberately.

When influenced by others, at some point the answers may reveal the true attribution of the desire to modify the appearance. A person unable to detail much of anything when asked these questions might have an immature understanding of the concepts involved and may be asked to think more about it, and then return when they have given it more analysis. Any patient who responds with "You're the doctor; can't you see it?" when asked what it is he or she wants to change will need further time to reveal himself or herself and may be best left to ponder why his or her request was turned down.

Persons who have a vague and idealized concept of what the surgery will do for them make poor patients especially if they anticipate a major change in lifestyle to be achieved after the procedure. If they voice that their new attractiveness will gain them riches, love, and power, they obviously have unrealistic expectations, and when the rare complication occurs or the result is less than expected, they can develop all sorts of reactive behavior, most of which is directed at the surgeon.

THE PSYCHOLOGICALLY FIT PLASTIC SURGERY PATIENT

Having a feature that has bothered one since puberty or since the self-image developed is part of what makes up the human psyche. It is the person's own rating of himself or herself when he or she looks in a mirror, sees himself or herself in pictures, or hears a casual remark about him or her not intended for their consumption. Wanting to change that feature can be a normal reaction and should be accompanied by expectations he or she will still be the same person when it is all over but without this deep-seated burden. Persons who were, however, ridiculed because of that feature and have developed immature coping mechanisms may still make good patients, but the degree to which they have altered their life due to shame and embarrassment cannot be determined by the average plastic surgeon. These types, if detected by the surgeon, may do well with referral to a professional counselor first and then undergoing the surgery once the coping mechanism has been dealt with.

It is normal to have some anxiety when the plastic surgeon first addresses the issue. These should fade as the consultation progresses. When the exact opposite occurs, and anxiety overtakes the interaction, a second appointment may be needed to find out the true motivation and whether or not the surgery should be done at this point. The best patients are relieved to hear the news that the surgeon has seen it all before, can give them the change in their appearance that they seek, and that the procedure is common.

It is also common as one ages to see features that remind oneself of one's parents at an older stage of one's life. Every plastic surgeon performing facial surgery has heard "I look just like my mother did in her fifties and I'm not going there." This motivation by itself can be considered realistic unless it is accompanied by other statements about the parental relationship, indications that it is more than the similar appearance that is at stake. Hints of maladjustment to the parental bonds may need some further investigation, but in general, this request is simple to understand and is often a normal reaction to aging in general.

Dealing with the ravages of pregnancy on the female figure is another frequent request for the plastic surgeon. Having a reasonable understanding of just how many stretch marks can be removed is key for a patient when they have occurred to a vast extent throughout the abdomen. Breasts that used to be perkier before nursing two to three or more children and now appear vacant of tissue can bother women who once thought that this was their best feature. Can both the abdomen and the breasts be addressed at the same operation? Yes, when the patient is young and healthy with no comorbidity and the anesthetic duration is reasonable.

But a patient who implores the surgeon to continue to add more and more procedures "while you're there, doc" may have a poor understanding of recovery and what will be involved. Television programs have glamorized the "makeover" and given many women false hopes that they can emerge from the operating room with a new face and a new figure in no time at all. Patients who are easily persuaded that it may not be in their best interest to have more than two procedures combined are good candidates for the surgery. Women who shop from surgeon to surgeon until they find one willing to spend an entire day operating on them head to toe can put themselves in dangerous and precarious postoperative conditions and should be counseled carefully on why they cannot accept breaking the "makeover" into stages.

Motivations for plastic surgery in men are addressed in detail in another chapter. The experienced surgeon will have encountered the situation more than once in his or her practice where a couple, husband and wife or partners, have asked to undergo simultaneous operations. This motivation is understandable when it is a question of both taking the time away from social and business situations and enduring the recovery period concurrently. Expectations of who can perform the act of cohort for the other is a question that should be met with understanding and realistically altered easily by the surgeon. Separating out the day of surgery so that one of the partners is clearheaded and mobile enough to care for the other should be met with acceptance, not protest. Ganging up on the surgeon or pushing the limits of what he or she thinks is appropriate may mean the couple should look elsewhere. Following the rules readily and understanding what the recovery will realistically involve indicate a couple that can have a satisfactory experience and accomplish exactly what they set out to obtain.

THE PSYCHOLOGY OF POSTOPERATIVE DISAPPOINTMENT

Malpractice cases can stem from many things, not just complications of the procedure itself. Cases where the surgeon misinterpreted the warning signs of infection and the patient developed heavy scarring afterward can bring contention over this to the door of the insurance carrier. Asymmetrical breasts after reduction or lifting will bring up questions of what went wrong. Regardless of the right or wrong answer, when questioned as to what happened, the way in which the surgeon approaches this patient can set the stage for mollification or retribution regardless of the answer.

But what about the instance where the surgeon is delighted with the results and the patient is not. Final outcomes may be acceptable to the professional because he or she avoided a complication and left the patient with no ongoing deficit of tissue or function. Yet the patient expected more and feels cheated, possibly to the point of wanting his or her money back. These delicate situations arise in the practice of every busy surgeon. Are these people who would have been better off not having the procedure in the first place? Did the surgeon fail to impart to them before the operation what to expect from the end result? Possibly.

Most often when the truth comes out and the surgeon is able to drill down to the root of this, it is because of a phenomenon unique to the practice of cosmetic surgery. One of the things these disappointed patients have in common is the admission, often with reluctance, that "No one noticed," which the surgeon might interpret as "They noticed but perhaps were being polite not to say anything."

When one paints one's house a strikingly different color, the neighbors will comment, perhaps too much, about what it did for the neighborhood. Cosmetic surgery patients can have the expectation that what they have paid for should get noticed just as much as a new hairstyle or a new handbag or a new coat of paint. When they hear nothing about their new look, they may try to blame things back on the surgeon. Suddenly, when the patient was expected to have a simple follow-up appointment after the surgery, perhaps 10 or 15 min in length, the surgeon finds himself embroiled in an emotional encounter seeking desperately to find out why his or her handiwork is underappreciated and accusations are flying. This is especially bothersome when the surgeon went to great lengths to analyze that this very patient was stable and properly motivated for the procedure requested.

In the business of facelifts, this is a puzzling, complex state of affairs. Getting the natural soft look, neither stretched too tight nor a dead give away that something was obviously "done," is the goal of most surgeons. But erasing every wrinkle, elevating cheek lines, and lifting brows to unnaturally high positions are in some instances the look patients are after. Is it because of what it says about their financial status? Paying exorbitant fees for a new appearance and not getting noticed for all that effort is not acceptable to some. Showing off what your cash horde can do is unfortunately what some patients seek. Just as unfortunate is the presence of many a good surgeon who is willing to participate in producing this satisfaction.

There are two types of patients who seek out breast enlargement, those who want no one to know and those who not only do not care who knows but who also seek to tell anyone who will listen about their new chest. Surgeons have known for decades that the types of placement of the breast implant can be varied enough to make things look natural or not. A large implant placed high on the chest wall and under the breast gland but not under the pectoral muscle can accentuate a rounded upper portion of the breast. It is as if the woman was wearing a push-up bra even when she was not. Astonishingly, after many decades of trying to avoid this look, surgeons are now finding young women who are asking to achieve just that because they prefer it. Social norms have changed so that now it is not only acceptable to have "fake boobs," but it is also desirable to let the world know you do indeed have implants.

Carefully counseling these requests for the look that seems counterproductive to the surgeon is necessary. The dilemma for the surgeon is whether or not to capitulate to the desire of the patient, or to hold fast to his or her own standards. When the surgeon says he will not participate in this request, the patient will shop around until he or she finds a surgeon who will, even if it means traveling distances to do so. The next time a patient comes through with this request, the surgeon may change his or her stance on the subject.

As testament to this problem, there are increasing numbers of malpractice claims, once considered nuisance claims, filed for the simple reason that "I didn't get the look I wanted!" While none of these simple demands wind up going the distance, that is, to a jury trial, there are, however, more and more cases where the surgeon capitulated to the demand for a more obvious look. After numerous surgical attempts to produce what the patient demanded, the surgeon instead wound up with an even unhappier patient, especially if along the way there was a significant complication. These demands are taken seriously by the insurance carrier, as are the accompanying calculations that a jury will feel more sorry for the patient or for the surgeon. Often there is no way to predict who will look more silly to them in the end in these types of cases.

THE FUTURE

All this would be an unnecessary discussion if only there was a tool that could correctly predict the ability of the surgeon to match what it is the patient wants, and what the surgeon needs to do to produce it. Detecting which patients are not yet ready for a cosmetic procedure or which patients will handle a complication with grace and dignity would be a welcome relief for many surgeons who have had to rely on gut instinct since the dawn of the specialty. Will such a simple test become available some day? Possibly, but the more important question is "when such a predictor arrives, will it be foolproof?" Every busy surgeon has memories of a patient who seemed certain to be able to go through a surgery with no problems, one who seemed psychologically fit as a fiddle. Yet this patient turned out to be exactly the opposite in the end, and the memories still make the surgeon restless when recalling it.

If it was easy and a computer could do it, then it would have been done by now. Unfortunately, human nature is complex; it is subject to the nuances of whims, the hurtful remarks of others, and lots of other external forces the surgeon will never know about. The human psyche can be unstable at one time, more stable at others. For now, surgeons will continue to rely on their own perceptions of their patients, skills learned over the years and the realization they may not always be capable of getting it right. Until that computer comes along that can predict postoperative behavior and satisfaction, the surgeon's gut reaction is all we will ever have.

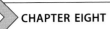

CHAPTER EIGHT

The Role of the Office Staff in Preventing Liability

The nurses and front office staff for any surgeon are the lifeline to the patients. The intimate role they play in direct contact with patients both before and after surgery cannot be overemphasized. Whether it is the first consultation or the first day after a complication, how they interact in both situations will be critical to the patient's perception of the surgeon, his or her skills and results. A single casual, aloof, or cold comment can send the wrong message at a critical time during the recovery phase, when the patient may be overtly concerned that he or she is not healing correctly or that something went wrong in surgery.

On the other hand, a caring, kind word or a warm touch can be all it takes to reassure patients that things are going in the right direction. A wise surgeon takes time to make sure that the right message gets sent by the entire staff at all times through training, review, and corrective action whenever the need arises. Keeping patients happy despite their own bad behavior and poor treatment of the staff can make the difference between anger diffused and anger brought to a plaintiff's attorney. The outcomes will be of course entirely different.

A surgeon can be the warmest, most charismatic soul, with adoring patients, but if his or her staff is hurried, stressed, and angry, early warning signs that the patient may not be happy with the surgical outcome could be missed. A patient who is already questioning why he or she chose a cantankerous surgeon will get a strong confirmation of their mistake when the staff is rude, coarse, and grumpy as well.

A split message, that "some of us care about you but the doctor doesn't", is still far better than the unified message that "none of us care about you at all". The flipside, perception of a doctor that cares a great deal whilst the staff couldn't care less, while not ideal, may still trump the worst scenario, no one gives a hoot. After all, rude treatment at general medicine clinics is rather legendary these days. Some patients simply become immune to it, not expecting anything more.

But the best alternative, where the truly warm and caring staff reflect the same behavior in the surgeon can go a long way to overcome complications, even severe ones, keeping the patient mollified and out of the tentacles of an aggressive attorney.

What happens in the exam room when the doctor is present can be overtly different than when the surgeon leaves the room. Every plastic surgeon has seen examples of this phenomenon. The fact is, what is communicated to the nurse can be an outpouring of concern held back from the surgeon so as not to appear to question or insult his or her work. The crucial next step is to make sure that this information gets passed on to the surgeon, just as a lab result or an X-ray would.

As a society in general, we often may feel constrained to speak out to authority figures, to admit that how we really feel inside is quite different than our outward appearance and our verbal presentation. Perhaps this is a generational condition, with older patients more prone to reticence than younger ones. Perhaps patients hold back in fear that the surgeon will abandon them if they voice their disappointment with the results. When the surgeon encounters a patient with chronic complaints, who never seems to accept the results, there can be a tendency to tune that patient out, possibly missing a key message that this is truly an unhappy patient and not just one prone to complaining. Experienced nurses often are the key to helping the surgeon identify the patients who may go on to become vindictive.

In some classic situations, this communication problem is simply gender related. Female patients at times may feel much more comfortable pouring out their concerns to another woman than to a man, especially if the surgeon is unapproachable and lacks warmth in interpersonal interactions. Failing to provide the female patient the time and opportunity to present her concerns to anyone can be a recipe for disaster. After all, how can anything be wrong when the surgeon does all the talking and leaves the room in a whirlwind with white coat flapping in his or her jet stream and the nurse totally absent from this scene? This type of surgeon does better only when he or she is followed by an unhurried, sympathetic nurse, be it male or female, with much more time on their hands.

How all these scenarios play out over time can be the key to what happens next, when the disillusioned, angry, and disgusted patient gives up on the doctor-patient relationship. Perceiving a patient's feelings and acting correctly on them should not be the sole domain of the surgeon. The best surgical practices have open staff relationships, dialog that freely flows uphill as well as down, and plans in place for dealing with tense, threatening situations as they arise.

These are the elements every surgeon should consider whether in a university setting, a multi-specialty clinic, employed at a hospital, or in solo private practice. Regardless of the practice type, every surgeon can use the staff to their advantage in preventing an angry patient from becoming a litiginous one.

TEAMWORK

Among all the other rules for the staff such as how to keep the chart up to date, filing of lab reports, and the like, another good idea is to determine who should have a presence in the exam room at a time when things may not be going in the right direction. This takes teamwork, when the signals are picked up that an appointment may not be the usual post-operative follow up exam with the typical happy patient.

An angry patient, demanding an explanation of what went wrong, needs more than a dressing change and a card for his or her next appointment. Having witnesses to what the patient communicates verbally and non-verbally to the surgeon in these situations should always be considered, especially if a staff member has already built a communication bond with the patient.

At the point where the angry patient has brought along relatives or friends who glare throughout the encounter or who make outright accusations and threats toward the surgeon, it is not only critical that the surgeon be accompanied by a staff member at all times but that what is said and played out should also be written down in the chart by him or her. This is no situation for a neophyte staff member.

A common mistake is for the surgeon facing this level of anger to hide the threats and implications from his or her staff. Perhaps, it is the need to deny that this relationship with the patient has disintegrated; perhaps, it is also the desire to keep the staff in the dark out of fear that they will "talk out of school" to others. Whatever the reason however, trying to keep the staff out of the mess can be completely counter-productive in most cases.

Surgeons may feel deeply embarrassed over patients' complications or angry themselves at the patient for contributing to them as well. In these encounters, a whole host of other internal emotions will arise. Thinking clearly and resisting the temptation to raise one's own voice can be challenging for the surgeon especially when fatigued or stressed by other issues.

With a team member in place it can be easier to avoid wallowing in the same mud with angry patients.

Witnessing and encountering these accusations as well as contributing to the conversation may indeed be a critical role for the nurse. However, if the surgeon intends his or her staff to participate as a witness only or as a referee in the discussion, how that role will be fulfilled should be arranged before the entrance to the exam room.

Often there may be one member of the office staff who has established some rapport. If so, he or she should be present and allowed to speak as well.

Front office staff as well as business staff all need to be alerted to the needs of this special patient. In his or her whirlwind of retribution, the patient may contact many of the staff, even polling them for their opinion on what went wrong. Failing to alert everyone on the team that this patient must be handled with care can contribute to a negative outcome. Some of the staff may already be aware of the tension, the demands, and the downward spiral. All of them should be on alert. Some offices even go so far as to put a special sign on the chart, such as a red star, making sure that everyone knows the special conditions needed.

With the entire team therefore working in unison to get the best outcome, eventually there should be a satisfied patient, one who goes on to achieve both physical and emotional healing.

COMMUNICATION

Patients often withhold their inner feelings from the surgeon but do not hold back with staff. It is therefore critical that a policy be in place to address such situations. Nurses can make good listeners, prone to nurturing and comforting. But if they are afraid to share what they know with the surgeon, or feel that since information was given in confidence and they should not pass it on, no favors for the employer have been done.

No surgeon ever wants to be breaking the bad news to the staff about a newly filed lawsuit only to hear them say, "We knew she would do it!" There should never be a surprise about anything at this point. Open communication both from the surgeon to the staff and vice versa should always be encouraged. The office environment should be unrestrained, such that this is not difficult for anyone no matter his or her status. No one should feel constrained from freely communicating what he or she has heard the patient say out of range of the surgeon's ears.

As soon as the angry patient reveals his or her plans such as obtaining a second opinion or that he or she will be contacting an attorney, this information needs to be passed on to the surgeon. Likewise, the surgeon should be in control of his or her emotions so as not to "shoot the messenger" when bad news is delivered. Staff members who gather outside the surgeon's office drawing straws to see who must go in and break the bad news will also most likely be less than supportive of the outcome. Staff who feel satisfied with a surgeon's misfortune have no place in the plastic surgery office. They will be the ones to poison the well whenever possible, no matter how loyal they seem.

POLICY CHANGES FOR THE ANGRY PATIENT

Once it has been established that there is the potential with a disgruntled patient for legal activity, basic planning needs to take place and some consideration for special attention for this patient should be taken into account. This might include simple changes such as altering when to bring the patient in for his or her appointments. It is critical that the surgeon has enough time to listen, think clearly, and work closely toward resolution in the exam room. If the schedule is tightly packed and a 10 minute time slot for this patient has become totally unreasonable, the staff should plan to bring the patient back within a few days. Clearing the clinical schedule for an hour or more, eliminating phone calls or other interruptions, and optimizing the patient's encounter is one action plan that may work to simply give the angry patients the satisfaction that they were "heard," and not brushed off.

Other plans include bringing the patient back at a time when the waiting room is empty, reducing the chance that this patient will encounter others and declare his or her disappointment with anyone willing to listen. Taking one's anger out in front of other patients in an attempt at retribution can occasionally occur and it should be anticipated. Most often it is wise to reduce any and all such encounters whenever the hostile patient is due for a visit.

AVOIDING THIS TYPE OF PATIENT IN THE FIRST PLACE

Every plastic surgeon will eventually encounter a patient he or she wishes they hadn't operated on. It is part of the profession, and extends to other subspecialists as well. But learning from one's mistakes should reduce the frequency of the need for personal soul searching and keep recurrent bad choices to a minimum.

The upside of keeping longstanding employees is the possibility that they can develop a sixth sense for who might become a problem patient. Nurses may see the patient in a different light on the first visit, hear things the surgeon doesn't, and have their own built-in receptors for warning signs. If the office environment is optimal, anyone, even the receptionist, should have the authority to come to the surgeon and freely discuss his or her concerns, especially before the patient signs up for an operation. The wise surgeon will listen openly at this point, recognizing that once the knife is put to the skin, the entire office has now accepted responsibility for what happens afterwards.

When the surgeon ignores this staff "barometer" and proceeds to operate on the patient anyway, if things go bad (as predicted), will the surgeon be abandoned by his or her staff, preferring to stand on the sidelines saying, "I told you so?" In a dysfunctional office, this may very well take place. A well functioning staff, however, will take all things into account and still support the surgeon in the postoperative care, no matter the urge to be smug and aloof.

WHAT THE OFFICE STAFF MUST NOT DO

The wise surgeon will also take steps to see that the office staff encounters with the patient are not only optimized but uniform as well. Codifying these patient care policies will never hurt one's practice. Ignoring them may ultimately cost the surgeon and runs the risk ultimately of dealing with it some day in court instead. Written staff policies on behavior only make good sense.

Under no circumstances should any staff be allowed to argue with a patient. While there may not be the need to go to the extreme dictum taken from the pages of customer service manuals such as "The patient is always right," when the patient is clearly wrong the situation must be diffused, not turned up to boiling. The ultimate extension of this is a written policy that any employee who openly argues with a patient may have an employment review and such negative encounters might be grounds for dismissal.

In the situation where the demanding patient wants an explanation for "what went wrong" from the staff, there is little room for anyone but the surgeon to answer this. All staff must be trained in this situation to politely defer to the surgeon, and refrain from voicing their own opinions or their version of what they think took place. Stoking the fires, rather than putting them out should be clearly grounds for review and even dismissal when needed.

If necessary, the surgeon might meet with the entire staff and ensure that one single voice is being heard, that everyone's viewpoint on what happened reflects that of the surgeon. Patients can be expert at polling any and all staff for their opinion. It is only good policy to be sure that these situations are not further confused or inflamed by a chatty opinionated staff.

It is not uncommon for the office staff at this point to have developed their own very negative feelings toward these patients. This can lead to avoidance, curt encounters, or just complete reticence when the patient comes back for an appointment. Behaviors such as these can then send a strong negative message to the patient at exactly the time the opposite message should be sent. Openly reviewing this with the staff before an unhappy, demanding patient's next encounter is far better than forever losing the patient at the worst possible time because of the staff's subconscious rejection of him or her entirely.

Staff should also be counseled to avoid making any effort to shield the surgeon from the angry patient. Many will try to set limits with the patient, hoping to reduce the surgeon's tension over these encounters, thereby also diffusing tension throughout the office. Likewise, the staff must resist the temptation to praise the surgeon, consciously or unconsciously, in front of the angry patient. There is no room at this point for adding salt to the wound by deifying the surgeon when the contrary evidence already exists on the patient's body. If this attitude is not discussed and stamped out or is perhaps even encouraged, trouble will not go away soon.

OTHER COMMON SENSE POLICIES
Privacy

Many surgeons over the course of their practice will encounter local personalities, famous for their contributions to the local society or whose employment has made them well known. Operating on the rich and the famous can have its own consequences. But no matter how these types of patients are handled by the staff, successfully or not, one policy makes good sense to have in place.

Many plastic surgeons now require their staff to sign a confidentiality agreement, stating clearly that revealing intimate details of who has had a procedure to their friends, reporters, or anyone outside of the office staff is grounds for dismissal. The mere presence of this policy sends a strong message to the surgeon's staff of a zero tolerance approach for breach of privacy. On the other hand, the surgeon employing such a policy with his or her staff must demonstrate the same commitment to not violate the patients' right to privacy themselves.

Staff surgery

Some plastic surgeons feel that operating personally on their own employees makes good sense. It builds staff loyalty through gifting a procedure, represents a profound employee benefit not obtainable in any other subspecialty, and can become an advertising source with a low price tag. Having that staff member available to meet with new patients, giving testimonials how easy the recovery was and how great he or she feels about the procedure can work wonders. But it makes good sense to have a written policy in place regarding how often they can return to the operating room for additional procedures, who is responsible for ancillary costs, and how a less than optimal result will affect one's employment. Treating each staff member fairly with a written policy spelling out these details is a must to avoid jealousy and recrimination among the staff.

On the other hand, what may seem like a terrific result to the surgeon can backfire when prospective patients don't see it in the same light. Super-sized breasts, revealed through unprofessional clothing, faces stretched beyond tight, and liposuction of every fat cell in the staff's body can be interpreted as a sign for some new patients to run away from this office. A wise surgeon thinks this through thoroughly and is not afraid to say no to a staff's request for more and more surgery, the same way as he or she would do with an unrealistic patient.

Personal appearance

This should not be a completely foreign concept to a successful plastic surgeon. But yes, the cleanliness of the office and in particular the staff has indeed caused some patients, when their wound became infected, to reach the wrong conclusion. With the names of drug resistant bacteria such as methycillin-resistant *Staph. aureus* on the lips of many patients, why would the surgeon let a slovenly appearing employee to cast a doubt, just from their casual approach to personal hygiene? Written policies are meant to not only alert employees to this potential but also back the surgeon up in the case of a frequent offender who needs dismissal from the staff because of his or her poor appearance. Patient acceptance of the facility and its employees will turn based on the satisfaction they have with the outcome. When they are have become truly disatisfied they will nitpick every detail to justify their unhappiness. The overall experience they have had can affect what they do next. A disheveled appearence of the staff will reinforce their new opinion that their outcome was caused by a surgeon who didn't really care about them, since he or she does not appear to care about the staff and their appearance.

SUMMARY

How the office staff of a plastic surgeon interacts with the patients can be a critical determinate of not just the success of the practice but whether or not the rare problem case will be attenuated successfully as well. The complex role that a surgeon plays in the practice, besides performing the operations successfully, must include among other key roles, the staff leader and the coach of their attitude and policies. All of these should be meshed successfully into a smooth-running machine that will not miss a beat when an unhappy patient returns. Scrutiny of the staff from time to time to ensure that they are prepared to handle these types of patients just makes good sense.

CHAPTER NINE

The Myths of the "No Risk," Minimally Invasive Office-Based Treatment

Much has been made of the advantages of using minimally invasive treatments to maximize the foot traffic into a plastic surgeon's waiting room. The easy to administer, high-volume injectible treatments should ideally amplify the exposure of the surgeon's repertoire to people who might not otherwise feel compelled to seek out a surgical procedure.

As predicted, they return again and again for more non-invasive treatments until eventually they satisfy their curiosity about a particular procedure asking for more information and a consult. By patiently treating their wrinkles and poor skin with easy to administer skin treatments and injectibles, the surgeon wins twice, doubling the chances that his or her income will benefit from this plan. The hope is that this ultimately creates a patient who stays in the practice for life, eventually having procedure after procedure. The theory sometimes works.

Traditionally, this focus on building long-lasting relationships with pateints was the domain of the plastic surgeon, until the non-surgical specialists such as dermatologists understood there was plenty of room for them to offer these treatments as well. As this segment for the manufacturers became saturated, however, they began to look beyond the traditional providers knowing that the only potential for growth was to make every single physician regardless of their specialty capable of offering injectibles in his or her practice. As attestations began to arise that the non-surgical physicians' incomes derived from these beauty treatments were far more than they had ever derived from history-taking and physical examinations, the market for these providers to become injectors went on to expand exponentially. As a result, it is now increasingly just as common to find botulinum toxin injections available at a family medicine office, as at the offices of a plastic surgeon or a dermatologist, where they were traditionally first offered.

It is also not uncommon to find all sorts of injectibles being proffered at health clubs, day spas, and parties administered by a Registered Nurse or just about anyone who can obtain the product, sometimes supposedly under the auspices of a person with an MD behind his or her name. But unfortunately, just as often the chances are that the physician whose name and license was used to obtain the product probably has never set foot in that health club or spa in his or her life, let alone evaluated the person receiving the injections.

This new paradigm, where there are no controls over who does what with cosmetic injections, has come about because of two factors. Few states yet regulate the performance of minimally invasive treatments. (As of this writing, only four states have laws pertaining to this.) Secondly, the more important part of the problem is that the manufacturers have denied responsibility for both regulating the training of the injectors (other than with a few marketing videos and brochures) and controlling whom they sell their products to. These companies have made a deliberate business decision not to control the end point distribution of their products. Thus, the arena of cosmetic injections has become a free-for-all when it comes to who has the best training for administering them, where they are available from, and how much the consumer pays for them.

The next myth, that with a little practice and experience any one can become specialized in minimally invasive treatments (with very few legal consequences) in fact probably has some truth to it. With a keen eye, some patience, and good record keeping, the ability to develop the skill-set needed to get predictable and successful results does not necessarily depend on the number of years spent in postgraduate training. Anyone can register for and take a weekend seminar on these injections. No one knows yet how steep this learning curve is, and the maxim that all it takes is experience is supported by the next myth that there are no legal, social, or ethical consequences to pay for mistakes made in this arena.

Contrary to all of this, however, is that in fact there are increasing numbers of lawsuits being filed over injectible and laser cosmetic treatments that lead to, in the least severe patient disappointment and beyond that serious disfigurement. Are these serious claims? Some could be categorized as frivolous or nonsensical. A few are, however, troubling because of the true permanent deformities that occurred, complications that unfortunately can happen even with experienced MDs holding the syringe or the hand piece.

So despite the myths to the contrary, there actually are some predict-able levels of side effects and complications for minimally invasive treatments. What fuels the myths is the belief that these treatments are free of *permanent effects*. That is, if the patient suffers in any way, as soon as the intended and unintended effects wear off in, say, 4 to 6 months, he or she will look as they did prior to the injection, no harm done.

The other problem with these myths is that they simply ignore that some of the substances now being injected are in fact semi–permanent to permanent and will not readily resolve by themselves in time if placed improperly. It is also assumed that these treatments are performed in a sterile fashion. But infections arising from contaminated needles and products can be permanently disfiguring with both permanent scars and soft tissue loss.

Clever attorneys have found that no matter how normal the patient looks once resolution from these complications has occurred, photographs of their distressed client suffering from the unusual appearance shortly after a treatment went awry, accompanied by a litany of their emotional sufferings, are all that it takes to squeeze a settlement out of the provider in time.

Beyond the injectible dilemmas, even larger problems occur with lasers and other energy based treatments, similarly when they are promised to be of low risk or even risk free, and significant complications arise after operator error and poor judgment.

The following list includes the reasons these claims continue to be filed in increasing numbers for these supposedly innocuous, minimally invasive office-based encounters.

TEMPORARY DISFIGUREMENT

The one well-known side effect of botulinum A treatments around the eyebrow is eyelid ptosis. The incidence is reported to be as high as 5% and the occurrence is usually within two weeks after the injection. The mechanism of ptosis is presumed to be extravasations or migration of the botulinum toxin from the injection site under the orbital septum, eventually paralyzing the levator palpebrae superioris muscle, albeit temporarily.

Patients who have experienced this have several things in common. It usually occurs unilaterally giving them a rather unusual look, somewhat akin to the effects of a minor cerebrovascular accident or stroke. Most of them, whether or not they were forewarned of this possibility in an informed consent document, are also highly emotionally distressed and fiercely angry about the occurrence.

While Iopidem eyedrops have successfully undone the side effect of lid ptosis in many patients, it is expensive and not every injector is aware of its availability. So while waiting for the return of the muscle function for a matter of months seems to be the only other option, reducing the emotional suffering the patient claims to be experiencing is also critically important to the provider who performed the errant injection.

In time, the normal appearance of the eyelid will return, and to date, there have been no reports of permanent facial muscle dysfunction from botulinum A. How long this return to normalcy will take is unpredictable but it is usually months not weeks. Some of these patients, especially those whose job depends on face-to-face meetings and being in the public's eye, feel they look hideous and will not go out of their house or go to work. Some have even reportedly been fired for failing to return to work at all for months. Those who do carry on their normal routines will not hesitate to condemn the provider publicly for causing the ptosis, an assault on one's reputation no physician wishes to have.

Once the lawyer has been contacted by the patient and the claim filed against whoever performed the treatment, the demands will include reparations for lost wages, emotional suffering and distress, and punitive awards for failing to provide appropriate informed consent. These claims will be based on charges of faulty technique in performance of the injection and a general violation of the standard of care, or what a reasonable physician with similar training would have done in like circumstances.

The standard informed consent document suggested for any botulinum injection includes written warnings of the possibility of asymmetrical results and lid ptosis. The length of time the distress over this appearance lasts however is not usually indicated on these documents, another point the aggressive attorney will make – if the patient had known about the length of the temporary disfugurment, he or she would of course never have given his or her consent.

In addition, some providers do not think it necessary to obtain a fresh consent form after the first one is signed, especially for patients who have received these injections up to three times a year or more and are very familiar with them. The opposite argument, however, is that memories are short and getting written consent for every subsequent injection will prove that the provider took this procedure seriously and was aware of the consequences of eyelid ptosis. Ultimately, it will be up to the patient and his or her attorney to prove what the standard of care was, and that the appropriate consent forms were on a par with those of the injector's peers who also provide this service.

ASYMMETRY FROM FILLERS

With hyaluronic acid based or other "filler" injections, the most common side effect is severe bruising which can last in some individuals for weeks. The potential for this should always be discussed with each patient on the first encounter, along with a reminder that aspirin or other anticoagulant usage should be discontinued for an appropriate length of time before the injection. Side effects from bruising should also be included in the informed consent documents. In fair skinned patients, hemosiderin deposits can have permanent effects on skin pigmentation when subjected to ultra-violet light during the recovery phase from the injections.

Besides bruising, there is the possibility of infection from a con-taminated injection needle or from a contaminated product itself. Skin loss after severe abscess formation can occur especially when antibiotic or drainage treatment is delayed. When infections cause permanent changes to skin contour and loss of subcutaneous fat, this can be fodder for filing a lawsuit against the person who performed the injection, claiming perma-nent disfigurement.

The most common complaint after any type of filler injection is unevenness and frank asymmetry. With longer lasting and even permanent substances being injected, any extreme difference from side to side will be grounds for discussion for some unhappy patients with a local plaintiff's attorney, especially if the injector did nothing to try to even out the prob-lem. As with botulinum induced eyelid ptosis, the demand will be for damages based on emotional distress over one's "hideous" appearance, even when it was temporary, and lost wages when the unsightly results meant staying home. Usually, by the time these patients get around to the lawyer, they have seen several other specialists and have a litany of additional treatments and charges. These will be passed along of course in the demand.

Hyaluronic acid treatments gone awry can be treated with medications as well. Hyaluronadase can be injected into the areas of unevenness or asymmetry, dissolving the product back into the other soft tissues or making it more absorbable. Just as with iopidem, when the allegations against the injector including failing to be aware of an "antidote" for the offending substance are made, the failure to at least consider the antidote will be a major trumped up charge by the attorney. Documenting in the chart that the physician was aware of these treatments but decided not to pursue them for a rational reason is essential when the unhappy patient returns and makes accusations of errors.

Many of these emotionally distressed patients will demand a refund. The willingness of the provider who created the asymmetry in the first place to stump up the cash in order to mollify this unhappiness depends on his or her moral indignation once such demands are made known. Waiting it out in a kind of medical-legal game of chicken, to or pay the demanding patient and move on with life, is a personal choice each provider will make, some resolved that it is simply a part of the cost of doing business.

When a physician suffers a string of these claims however the malpractice insurance carrier will be taking a hard look at a physician's risk profile through their underwriting department. No matter how long that provider has loyally paid the policy premiums, taking on uncertain risks and performing outside of the standard of care eventually may cause cancellation of the policy and searching for a new insurance provider.

SCARRING FROM LASER AND PHOTOTHERAPY TREATMENTS

The plethora of treatments for the correction of skin aging and sun damage can seem overwhelming to the casual observer. IPL (Intense Pulsed Light) for reducing brown spots and peeling the skin, photoelectric treatments for tightening the collagen layers, lasers for skin rejuvenation and hair removal, the list goes on and on. And so does the interesting ways these procedures can get the surgeon and/or the staff into trouble.

For the purpose of this chapter, all skin treatments that require a power source and an operator are lumped under the banner of "energy based therapy."

While none of the machines involved is completely idiot-proof, the manufacturing company whose sales staff depends on moving these products would have the physician think so. If it has a dial to increase or decrease the delivery of the end point to the skin, eventually someone will be confused, mistaken, or simply ignorant, and trouble will ensue.

There is an age-old principle in plastic surgery, a paradigm that will generally serve the surgeon well: "You can't insult the skin from both sides and get it to heal."

Unfortunately not everyone adheres to this. Cases continue to be filed against surgeons where the wide undermining of the skin during a facelift was followed, in the same procedure, with a machine-generated treatment to the dermis from the skin side. The resulting large necrotic patches of neck and facial skin will never go on to look normal no matter how many subsequent surgeries are done. The new paradigm therefore should be: "If it has a plug it also has the potential to be a problem."

The number one complaint from patients who signed up for laser hair removal is that it didn't work. This is closely related to the number of reasons for the filing of a lawsuit after laser hair removal. The patient went back to the surgeon's office or the medi-spa or the technician and wanted a refund or an additional treatment at no charge.

Here's where the rationale for taking the unhappy patient into the treatment room for another round of blasting away with the machine gets confused. Rather than suspect that the lack of response was possibly due to the timing of the 120 day hair cycle, or the light color of the patient's hair, or that this is a patient for whom the treatment will not be successful, what is seen too often is that the next treatment is simply done at higher power settings. The thinking is that the settings were probably not right the first time. In the unfortunate patients whose skin does not tolerate this new burst in energy, the resulting second degree burns will cause them to regret forever the day they decided to try to become hairless. These claims are arising too frequently to be ignored as just accidents, and there is little excuse for this occurrence.

Hypertrophic, hyperpigmented burns in the mons pubis, the lower extremity, the upper lip and covering the back are difficult to defend. Suggesting to a jury that this was the result of defective machinery and not a poor decision made by the operator will do little to get anyone out of the jury's scorn. Unfortunately, in most of the cases, the decision to turn up the power was made by an employee of the entity, whether it was a medi-spa or the physician's own office, and almost never with the input of the physician or someone else in charge. In some cases, the medical director of the medi-spa had never met the technicians much less supervised their work. Imagine then the surprise when he or she is suddenly named in a subpoena for these horrific looking scars that can never be improved. If it has a plug, then eventually it will be a problem.

So what is the wise plastic surgeon to do? That depends on how much supervision of staff he or she decides to take on. Delegating the tasks of using the "plug-in" machinery may extend the ability of the physician to be in two places at once. Teaching the nurses in one's office to do injections on the face will certainly increase the office income, but does it also increase the risk? That question must be asked internally of everyone who decides to take on the use of physician extenders.

As teaching courses for these machines exist, even if they are offered by the manufacturer rather than an independent non-biased source, not only should any staff using the machine go to these classes one from time to time but also the certificate of such attendance must be available for a jury to see some day. "On the job" training rather than continuing medical education that eventually allows these incidents to happen can be very problematic to defend in court.

FAILURE TO DO A "TEST PATCH" FIRST

No one in their right mind manufacturing or selling their own energy based treatment machines would fail to protect themselves from the potential to misuse these devices. Lasers, that if used incorrectly could produce corneal or retinal damage, have strongly worded warnings about the use of eye protection. Similarly, many of these also come with seldom-heeded warnings to perform a test spot on each patient's skin before both parties commit to a full treatment. If the test is done on skin adjacent to the hairline or another inconspicuous area and it turns hyper-pigmented or scarred in some way, then direct excision of the tested skin can be easily performed leaving an innocuous scar and hopefully one which will fade in time. The patient and the surgeon have learned not to proceed to a procedure that will run the high risk of unsightly scars or pigmentation and the contract is ended.

Too often, the decision to get a skin treatment is made somewhat impulsively, especially if the treatment is being pushed as one that is easy to recover from, such as a "lunch-time" fix, or just a matter of a few days of recovery before they look better. For certain skin types, this may be true. But for dark skinned clients this may be totally erroneous, not only with longer healing times but also potentially with permanent pigmentation changes. Impulsive shopping for shoes will not result in anything but some lost time taking them back if the buyer is disappointed. Impulsively having one's entire face treated with an energy based machine means that there is no going back to the return counter when the skin becomes irregular, blotchy, uneven, and of a different color permanently.

As the procedure is sold hard as being readily available and the technician has no one waiting, the pressure to do the whole face procedure and

skip the test patch will be driven by the need to keep the machine producing income and to capture the impulsive shopper. A test patch will frighten
some potential patients into thinking clearly and will be seen as causing
unnecessary worry for others whose skin might be the right type to simply
skip the test altogehter. The ethics of this decision, to follow the
manufacturers' recommendations to perform a test patch on all patients
(and risk losing many patients needlessly), is unfortunately not even considered by many of those who use these machines to make a living.

When it is time to face the fact that a claim has been filed for scarring
or pigmentation irregularities or usually both, the manufacturer will simply
note that their recommendations were not followed and they therefore
have no vicarious liability. They will point to the section in their instruction manual that notes that these are needed on all patients and then they
will file for release from the claim immediately after that.

When asked why the recommendations were not followed, the defen-
dant(s) in a suit who caused permanent scarring will have a hard time coming
up with a rational explanation for ignoring the instruction manual. The only
hope for a claim like this is to defend it on the basis of the standard of care,
that is, what others using the machine were doing in the same circumstances.
To be effective, the defendant's expert witness had better also have used the
machine successfully over and over again on the same type of skin.

Blaming the results on the patient and his or her failure to follow
instructions can occasionally work with some juries, but will backfire on
others. Why take the chance? A good policy demanding that dark skinned
individuals always get tested first will mean that the risk one might get
nailed by an angry jury may never take place. Even better is to be able
to successfully claim that test patches were always performed on everyone
as a matter of policy.

THE ETHICS OF LOW RISK TREATMENTS

Given the high costs of obtaining injectible products, it should
surprise no one that the temptation to cut a few corners is ever-present.
Botulinum toxins must be diluted before being administered. Following
the package insert still allows for flexibility as to the potency and strength
of the substance being inhected. Over-diluting the active ingredient but
charging full price as a normal dilution method will stretch the
wholesale cost out, especially if one doesn't care that some or many
patients will feel that they didn't quite get what they had asked for. Ethical

providers will resist this temptation. For others the temptation to profit from cheating things a bit is just too strong.

Add to that the physicians' constant barrage of e-mail, mail, and phone enticements to buy these injectibles at cut-rate prices from suppliers based outside of the United States. Can one ethically inject a substance that is not manufactured under the FDA's guidance and always get away with it? There is no doubt some have done so. Some plastic surgeons have failed to resist, when they have been suffered more than just embarrassment when they have to come clean and admit their transgressions.

There is little in medicine that is "can't miss." The myth of these "low risk" treatments is that they are essentially foolproof because the result is temporary. This seductive reasoning is hard to dismiss when the sales forces of large multinational companies perpetuate it while urging their products onto the hard working doctor. If it sounds too good to be true, then it probably is. Too many times the physician will be wringing their hands over what they learned about the no-risk treatment was unfortunatley the hard way.

Another critical mistake made when using these treatments through physician extenders is the failure to ensure that their license was current and that they were operating within the scope of that license (see Chapter 13.) Can medical assistants give injections? In some states yes, under the supervision of a physician. In other states, the answer is quite different. Can an aesthetician with a cosmetology license use a powerful laser? In most states it is unclear. As of the writing of this book in 2010, only four states have taken on the task of who should be doing what with which machine under what circumstances. It is up to the physician directing all this orchestration of nonsurgical treatment to know the laws, abide by them ethically, and take no chances.

Nothing in medicine is without risk as has been proven time and again. Risk that can be predicted is acceptable and can be insured. Myths cannot be insured. As they are often self-propagating until debunked, myths should also not be the basis for hard selling anything to an unsuspecting patient who then believes that what he or she is about to get is totally risk-free.

CHAPTER TEN

Claims Arising from Medi-Spas

Opening and managing a medi–spa may seem simple enough for surgeons who have run their own practice for years. Both require initial financial outlays, personnel decisions, policy and procedure manuals, and treatment guidelines. The only major differences at first glance might include stocking a large inventory of retail products and hiring enough people to manage the volume of customers beating a path to the door.

While this formula seems rather simple, it is not without medical-legal hazards. Common misbeliefs abound when it comes to the risks involved. The expansion of the surgery practice to a business that primarily exists to make a profit from volume based treatments and the sale of products presents many more opportunities for things to go wrong than a surgical office standing by itself. The odds are that running the medi-spa is far different than anything the surgeon has ever been trained for. Labor laws, business insurance, premises liability, and inventory protection are just a few of the pitfalls a surgeon can fall into as "The Practice" soon morphs into "The Salon."

Partnering with a business owner who brings the skills and expertise of the spa or salon industry along may be the safest way to get it right the first time. While it might mean a larger cash outlay at first, it might also help to avoid the frequent mistakes that surgeons make as they try themselves to understand the medi-spa environment. The problems in maintaining a partnership can also bring new stress to the business, especially when more expansion is needed to keep ahead of the competition and meet demand. The businessman may understand only the sales aspects whereas the surgeon may have a wary eye on the risks of the medical treatments. Quite possibly, neither of them would have planned at all for a catastrophe that could implode the entire operation.

Initially, from a risk standpoint, the medi-spa seems almost too good to be true. With a little advertising and a little luck, the clientele should consist of high volumes of female clients who desire to look younger, with better skin and healthier lifestyles. The ambience and service should bring them back for more. Treatments such as minimally invasive peels and other "low risk" abrasions with short recovery times abound for this group of women. These are essentially skin cleansing and beautifying applications with rapid recovery times, typically considered non-invasive and frequently are performed by an aesthetician.

But when the more invasive treatments are added, the potential for harm expands, despite the presence of a medical director, even one who remains "on-site" during all business hours. Only by undertaking a thorough evaluation of the wide range of risks involved with every treatment can the surgeon be completely protected. Ideally, this decision is made during the early planning stages and the start up of the spa, not after the firm is hit with a major disaster. The clear distinction of the use of new technologies where appropriate by registered nurses rather than medical assistants or aestheticians must be understood and rigidly adhered to in avoiding risk.

Even though the side effects from an invasive treatment can be predicted when administered by a professional with appropriate training, unanticipated complications can still occur even to the most experienced physicians. It is when these treatments are in high demand and the staff short-handed that things can get out of control. Bending the rules, breaching the policy and procedure manual, and violating state and local laws seem to be at the root of most of the disasters that have come to light in this industry.

For their own greatest protection, the owners of the medi-spa should be considering coverage in several basic areas, each needing a distinctly worded and separate liability policy, but all often sold in a package over and above the surgeon/owner's own malpractice policy. The following areas are the most common source of inadequate coverage for physicians exposed to liability in the medi-spa.

APPROPRIATE LICENSING AND TRAINING OF THE STAFF

All sorts of lasers and a wide array of other light or radio frequency machines are marketed as nearly foolproof ways to tighten the skin, reduce wrinkles, burn away age spots, and remove hair permanently. In most instances, this is very achievable. But if it has a power cord, it also has the ability to be misused or misapplied by an employee with no formal certification or training.

Liability claims for damages from the actual malfunctioning of these machines are rarely seen; the majority of claims for damages arise instead from totally preventable situations, almost all of them involving operator error. In the medi-spa, many-to-all of these treatments are performed by staff and not the physician, therefore it is up to the medical director to ensure that "under the supervision of a medical professional" means just that. Thousands of these treatments are undertaken by the staff regularly with the clients' presumption that the physician provided appropriate direction and legal coverage. In addition, many states now have regulations regarding what level of medical professional can use each of these types of machines and how strictly the physician supervision must be adhered to.

But settings that are not checked, training that was hurried and incomplete, and distractions at the time the treatment hand piece is picked up all can contribute to the injuries that occur when the machine is misused. Lawsuits arising from these situations usually are preceded by inattention, fatigue, lack of communication, under-staffing, and staff advancement and promotion with inadequate credentials and training.

When a complication arises from one of these treatments, the finding that the employee who administered it did not have proof of training, a certificate verifying they are fully trained to use it, and a current state license makes defense of the claim virtually impossible. All too often in these claims, the situation arose when over-worked employees gave "on the job" training to less experienced or non-licensed junior staff. Often the medical director has no knowledge of the "handover" but when the claim comes to fruition, he or she will still be held accountable. The deepest pockets will have to face the music. Without any insurance at all to cover this situation, the catastrophic results can ruin even the best-run businesses.

To cover this situation, there must be regular checks and balance in place to be sure that every licensed employee has a current certificate from an appropriate agency on file. Expired licenses can and will be discovered and can ruin the defense of a case in some instances.

Failure to keep on file the proof of training for each and every employee using any of the treatment machines is also a very black hole that will be difficult to crawl out of in the event of a claim.

The medical director's responsibility then is not just to bolster the image of the salon but, more importantly, to maintain that training of all employees is documented and current and to ensure that no one oversteps their bounds.

MEDICAL DIRECTOR'S ADDED PROTECTION

Underwriters hate unknowns, and in fact the entire industry is based on the predictability of all known and theoretical risks. In the past, as the typical beauty salon or lightly delineated "spa" began to take on more risk by adding complex medical procedures, the liability industry found that the old paradigms of risk assumption were no longer valid. This included the acceptance that there would be occasional claims for chemical burns from hair and scalp treatments, unexpected results from minor treatments, and the usual premises claims for slips, trips, and falls.

Embracing the new and increasingly more complex treatments in these spas meant that underwriting had to adapt to the new reality although with many new and misunderstood risks and unpredictability. This led to difficulty in finding appropriate pricing of policies and eventually reductions in coverage due to confusion over these issues.

Gradually, however, as the industry matured and more complex medical treatments were added, the insurance industry developed paradigms to keep up. These have now been formulated on two key presumptions: that the scope of services is known and carefully delineated and that the training and certification of the providers are qualified and enforced by a licensed professional whose own training is verified.

Therefore, the liability coverage for the medical director must consist of not only his or her own malpractice policy but also a second policy that provides specific protection for the acts of others performed under the direct supervision of that insured physician. These should be two separate and distinct policies. It is a mistake too often made that when hiring the medical director, the owners of the spa will automatically get his or her malpractice insurance to cover the entire staff. The fallacy is usually not discovered until it is too late, after the filing of a subpoena for malpractice.

In some instances the liability policy for the role of staff supervision by the medical director is simply an endorsement or rider added onto the medi-spa's own malpractice coverage. This is sometimes organized in such a fashion because at times the organization stands to benefit most from the relationship and therefore simply adds the coverage as a way of extending courtesy to the surgeon for his or her efforts. The surgeon must, however, still maintain his or her own treatment policy not only for direct patient care outside the medi-spa but also within the entity itself. This can become exceptionally important when two separate policies exist and they have been obtained through separate companies each with its own underwriting principles. Who covers what should be spelled out clearly so as to avoid confusion, mistrust, and ill will when the first claim arrives to upset everyone involved.

Pricing for the supervision policy is determined on the assumption of the technical skills and licensing of the employees being supervised as well as the degree of complexity of the procedures being performed by them. The closer these treatments come to the invasive rather than non-invasive nature the higher the price of course. It is ultimately the responsibility of the underwriters to calculate and assume the "knowns" rather than the "unknowns" in the medi-spa.

PRODUCT LIABILITY

Product sales directly to the consumer constitute a huge portion of the profits in most medi-spas. Typically these are "resale" items, meant to be specifically dispersed from a licensed facility, with the name of the known producer of each item clearly labeled on the product. Correct directions for the use of the product therefore will be printed on the container and any injury arising from the use of these chemical ingredients is typically the responsibility of the producer and not the seller.

These relationships change drastically for the medi-spa that takes any product from any producer and re-labels it with its own name and/or logo. Now the responsibility for any injury arising from the chemical ingredients will be directed at the owner of the label. Many of these plaintiff's claims will also name the original manufacturer once that becomes known. But it is unlikely as the claim procedes that the medi-spa and its medical director will be soon dropped from the proceedings no matter what the damages involved are. Legal wrangling over the implied responsibility for damages in such an instance can last years, not months.

Additional claims will inevitably arise if the medi-spa's employees direct the clients in the "off label" use of any product. These claims are defensible but take time and money to work their way to conclusion and will inevitably also name the medial director as the defendant in the process.

Thus, any liability policy for the medi-spa must also include product liability coverage. Where this becomes a problem is when the medi-spa takes on its own labelling without expanding the coverage for such new-found exposure.

EMPLOYMENT PRACTICES EXPOSURE

Coverage for claims emanating from disgruntled employees for such things as sexual harassment, wrongful termination, and all types of discrimination must always be provided, especially when there are increasing numbers of employees being added to the busy medi-spa. While typically most medical offices these days are well aware of the need to secure such coverage, when the surgeon changes the practice into a medi-spa, and adds a new name to the facility, the old policy might typically only provide coverage for the physician's practice and deny coverage for the new entity. It is far better to find that there was a discrepancy in coverage before a claim is filed by a former employee than when it arrives on the doorstep by subpoena after the name change.

DIRECTORS AND OFFICERS

Once the medi-spa becomes an entity and not the surgeon's practice, other exposures can occur. Coverage for any director's misstatements, or acts of omission or commission in carrying out the duties as a director, must be included in a separate policy. If the entity then also develops a Board of Directors, this policy must clearly cover them as well, spelling out the usual deductibles and limits of coverage. Ultimately, the responsibility for this coverage will always fall on the medical director as well as any other owners. Presuming that the coverage of the surgeon's office also applies to the new entity is a dangerous assumption and may lead to unnecessary and avoidable exposure.

In some markets in the United States, the bundling of several of these risk policies can be obtained so that a single policy covers employee practices exposure, product liability, and director's and officer's policies under one umbrella. Whether this reduces the overall price over and above the cost of each policy being written separately depends on the nature of the local market and the level of competition among underwriters in that region.

EMPLOYEE THEFT

In the ideal world, this would be an important part of a medi-spa's insurance package that could be extinguished. But this is not an ideal world and no one is above temptation, and in some spas, there is a general policy that all employees are encouraged to use the spa's products. What better testimony to give to potential clients/users than the fact "we all use it here and love it." This policy unfortunately can breed a "help yourself" attitude and create significant inventory shrinkage, as employees help themselves without the notion of it being a theft. After all it was encouraged. The next step is taking a few to give away at Christmas, and then on to supplying a few friends and family.

But the real threat to inventory, especially when it is poorly managed, is the employee who figures out that reselling the product at retail prices to his or her friends is suddenly a lucrative way to add to his or her meager earnings after deductions.

The best advice? Carefully control product inventory levels. Make a policy that still encourages the use of the products by the employees at no charge but registers each and every bottle, tube, or box with the employees taking it home and each time they do so. The amounts being charged to a write-off detected this way may ultimately be shocking. And finally, do not fail to have an insurance policy that will cover the cost of theft of large quantities of product right out from under the owner's nose. How often this occurs is probably unknown, but who cares to find out too late that they were suckers all along?

CONCLUSIONS

There are multiple risks inherent in developing and managing a medi-spa, that is, besides the inherent risk of losing money and ultimately experiencing a business failure. Working hard to make the enterprise successful also means realizing the inherent liability risks of the undertaking and successfully developing strategies for complete avoidance of them.

Any physician being asked to take on the position of medical director of an already ongoing medi-spa must know as well how much added risk he or she is going to be exposed to. All too often, the negotiations for this position involve only the compensation packages, the hours to be provided on the premises, and the number of employees to be supervised. It is all too often the mistake of the newly minted medical director to assume that the current surgical liability policy will cover the additional exposures as well. Accepting this position without a full calculation of the medi-spa's coverage for the director can be a set-up for disaster once the first claim arrives. A wise surgeon realizes these potential pitfalls and will get professional evaluations of the coverage or gaps in such setups before he or she completes the agreement.

CHAPTER ELEVEN

What Every Emerging Surgeon Should Know About Medical Liability

GENERAL CONSIDERATIONS

A plastic and reconstructive surgeon practicing in the United States in the 21st century will find it virtually impossible to end his or her career unblemished by a claim of malpractice. Whoever does so is certainly the rare exception. This, however, is not the place to review the pathogenesis of the single-most overriding socioeconomic issue of the medical profession in our time. What is called for are some clear, cogent, and immediately applicable guidelines which, if followed, should certainly reduce the probability of your involvement.

Well over half the claims in plastic surgery are preventable. Most are not based on technical faults, but rather on failures of communication or patient selection criteria. Patient selection is the ultimate inexact science. It is a mélange of surgical judgment, gut feelings, personality interactions, the surgeon's ego strength, and regrettably, economic considerations. The following article will hopefully help you with this aspect of your practice while choosing your patients for elective aesthetic surgery. Communication, on the other hand, is the sine qua non of building a doctor-patient relationship. Unfortunately, the ability to communicate well is a personality characteristic that cannot be readily learned in adulthood. Regardless of how brilliant the mind or deft the hands, someone who appears to be cold, arrogant, or insensitive is far more likely to be sued than one who relates to people at a "human" level.

It is highly unlikely that any surgeon will commit not a single error in their career. It is, however, entirely possible to alter the subsequent outcome of an error by adhering to a few simple rules.

STANDARD OF CARE

Malpractice is defined in legal lexicon as "treatment which is contrary to accepted medical standards and which produces injurious results in the patient." Although most medical malpractice actions are based on laws governing negligence, the law recognizes that medicine is an inexact art and that there cannot be absolute liability. Thus, the cause of action is usually the "failure of defendant/physician to exercise that reasonable degree of skill, learning, care, and treatment ordinarily possessed by others of the same profession in the community." In the past, the term *community* was accepted geographically, but this is no longer true. Now, on the supposition that all doctors keep up with the latest developments in their field, *community* is generally interpreted as the "specialty community." The standards are now those of the specialty, without regard to geographic location. This is usually referred to as *standard of care*.

Standard of care has special implications in plastic surgery; it is a specialty that encompasses many variations to achieve the same end. Thus, to a certain extent, the plastic surgeon has more latitude than do other surgeons because we have other ways to resolve the problem; thus no single method is absolute standard of care.

WARRANTY

The law holds that by merely engaging to render treatment, a doctor warrants that he or she has the learning and skill of the average member of his or her specialty and that he or she will apply that learning and skill with ordinary and reasonable care. This warranty of due care is legally implied; it need not be mentioned by the physician or the patient. However, the warranty is for service and not for cure. Thus, the doctor does not imply that the operation will be a success, that results will be favorable, or that he or she will not commit medical errors that are due to lack of skill and care.

One of the by-products of technology and the crunch of competition is the increasing popularity of "imaging devices." Although useful in planning craniofacial operations, these devices are now often used as inducements to aesthetic surgery. If a surgeon cannot deliver what was created on a computer screen, he or she may face a breach of warranty action. To a lesser extent, the same is true of showing pictures of *only* great results or enthusiastic testimonial statements of former patients. I strongly advise the use of a carefully worded disclaimer, written by legal counsel, for anyone who wishes to use an imaging device in patient consultation. If patient photographs are used, they should represent both excellent and only fair results to avoid an implied warranty.

INFORMED CONSENT

For centuries, Anglo-Saxon common law has respected an individual's right to the integrity of his or her person; any authorized "harmful or offensive touching" technically has constituted battery. Thus, a physician who treats a person without that person's consent is usually guilty of battery.

Since the term "informed consent" has become such an important, and often misunderstood, issue, we think it useful to clarify the meaning and application of this element in your practice.

How does informed consent differ from routine consent? In the former, the patient had sufficient understanding of the nature, purpose, and risks of the procedure to make an intelligent decision to accept or reject the procedure. Obviously, in discussing the risks, a certain amount of discretion must be employed. Is this consistent with "full disclosure" of facts necessary for informed consent? The emphasis is on the word *informed*. While attempting to define the yardstick of disclosure, the courts divide medical and surgical procedures into two categories:

1. Common procedures, which incur minor or very remote serious risks (including death or serious bodily harm), for example, the administration of antibiotics
2. Procedures involving serious risks, for which the doctor has an "affirmative duty to disclose the potential of death or serious harm and explain, in lengthy terms, the complications that might possibly occur"

Affirmative duty means that the physician is obliged to disclose, on his or her own, without waiting for the patient to ask. It is the patient, not the physician, who has the prerogative of determining his or her best interests. Thus, the physician is obliged to discuss with the patient the therapeutic alternatives and their particular hazards.

How much explanation, and in what detail, are dictated by a balance between the surgeon's feelings about his or her patient and the requirements of the law. You need not, in the words of a justice of the U.S. Supreme Court "engage in an orgy of open-minded disclosure." It is simply not possible to tell all patients everything that can happen without scaring them out of their surgery. Rather, as the law states, the patient must be told the most probable of the known dangers and the percent of that probability. The rest may be disclosed in general terms while reminding the patient that he or she also has a statistical probability of falling down and hurting himself or herself that very same day.

Obviously, the most common complications should be volunteered frankly and openly, and their probability, based on your personal experience, also should be mentioned.

In summary, although it may seem the ultimate platitude, the best way to stay out of trouble is to be honest, warm, and compassionate. If you use common sense and behave toward the patient as you would want another physician to behave toward your spouse, it is highly unlikely that you will have need of this information.

Unfortunately, in the current "state of the art," any or all of this information is wasted unless you document it. There is an eleventh commandment: Write it down!

THE THERAPEUTICS OF FULL INFORMED CONSENT

Up to this point informed consent has only been described in a legal sense, and nothing has been noted about its therapeutic effects. Simply stated, all this means is that the very act of disclosure will result in less anxiety, increased trust in the integrity of the physician, a smoother clinical course, and better understanding should anything go awry.

Some surgeons are reluctant to use consent forms, which explain possible negative outcomes, on the theory that calling attention to a long list of potential complications heightens the patient's unspoken anxieties unnecessarily. Ideally, the informed consent session should be viewed as an opportunity to dispel uncertainty, allay anxiety, and help fill the gap between the patient's ignorance and the physician's supposed omnipotence. By the "sharing of uncertainty," the physician can transform a potentially adversarial relationship into a "therapeutic alliance." In many therapeutic situations, the patient's principal defense mechanism against uncertainty is to endow the physician with a certain omnipotence. Thus, a relationship evolves in which the patient is totally dependent on the doctor, both physically and emotionally. If an unfavorable outcome shatters the "magic," the disillusionment may not only increase the patient's dependent state, but also may lead to refusal to accept prior knowledge of such an outcome or even to assume partial responsibility for self-care.

The surgeon should try to dispel any fantasies or unrealistic expectations before treatment begins. In practical terms, this problem could be addressed during the informed consent session. Consider, for example, the following two statements:

1. "Here is a list of complications that could occur during your treatment (operation). Please read it carefully and sign it. If you don't understand anything, ask me."

2. "I wish I could guarantee you that there will be no problems during your treatment (operation), but that wouldn't be realistic. Sometimes there are problems that cannot be foreseen, and you need to know about them. Please read about them, and let's talk about it."

In the second statement, the physician has reduced his or her omnipotent image in the patient's mind to that of a more realistic and imperfect human being who is facing, and thus sharing, the same uncertainty. The implication is clear: "We—you and I—are going to cooperate in doing something to your face/body that will make you better, but there are no guarantees on how you will respond. How you heal is as individual to you as the color of your hair and eyes."

In an effort to ease anxiety, a good physician may seek to reassure the patient and, in so doing, may over-reach and create not only unwarranted expectations but an implied guarantee.

1. Don't worry about a thing. I've taken care of hundreds of cases like yours. You'll do just fine.

2. "Barring any unforeseen problems, I see no reason why you shouldn't do very well. I'll certainly do everything I can to help you."

Again, in the second statement, the doctor is gently deflating the patient's fantasies down to realistic proportions while remaining reassuring and simultaneously helping the patient to accept reality.

The therapeutic objective of informed consent then should be to replace some of the patient's anxieties with a sense of participation and some "control." This strategy strengthens the therapeutic alliance between the patient and the physician. The patient will realize that the doctor is concerned and will do his or her part but is not GOD.

THE PSYCHODYNAMICS OF PATIENTS' ANGER

It is entirely appropriate for patients to feel a sense of bewilderment and anxiety, especially when elective surgery does not go smoothly. The borderline between anxiety and anger is very tenuous, and the conversion factor is uncertainty—the fear of the unknown.

How do we cope with uncertainty? Blaming someone else places the responsibility elsewhere and gives one a sense of "control," which, however inappropriate, is easier to cope with psychologically. A patient frightened by a postoperative complication, uncertain about the future, may gain a distorted sense of security by blaming the physician. The natural consequence of this distortion, then, is, "if it *is* the doctor's fault, the responsibility is the doctor's to correct."

The patient's distorted perception may clash head-on with the physician's understandable anxieties and wounded pride. The patient blames the physician, and he or she, in turn, becomes defensive. It is at this critically delicate juncture that the physician's reaction can set in motion, or prevent, a chain of reaction.

The physician must make a supreme effort to put aside feelings of disappointment, anxiety, defensiveness, and hostility that are natural to all of us when we are attacked. The physician must understand that he or she is probably dealing with a frightened patient who is using anger to gain "control" of the situation. The entire mood and subsequent developments can be changed by whatever understanding, support, and encouragement seem appropriate to the situation.

The perception by the patient that you understand the uncertainty and will join with him or her to help conquer it may be the deciding factor in whether or not the patient's next move is to seek legal counsel. When faced with someone who is upset or angry, it is best to remain silent and let that person talk about the problem. Only respond with noncommittal comments such as "yes" or "uh-huh" until the emotionally charged patient has calmed down. The technique of attentive silence often defuses angry people. Once the angry speaker has finished expressing his or her dissatisfaction, it is best to calmly ask the speaker to reiterate part of the message, even though you fully understood it. The request for additional information or explanation reinforces in the speaker's mind the importance you attach to the message.

One of the worst errors in dealing with angry or dissatisfied patients is to try to avoid them. Although this is an understandable reaction, it is easily the surest way to hasten the arrival of a summons and complaint. As difficult and stressful as it may be, the more you talk and *listen* to that patient, the more likely you are to avoid converting an incident into a claim. If you assume that at least 50 percent of the effort necessary for effective communication is your responsibility, you will successfully diffuse the ticking time bomb. It is necessary to actively participate in the process rather than follow your natural instincts and run away or hide.

PATIENT SELECTION

The growing popularity of aesthetic plastic surgery has, unfortunately, created a carnival-like atmosphere in which advertising by unqualified practitioners is only one aspect. In this climate, it becomes imperative to establish clear criteria of patient selection; without these, there will be an inevitable parallel increase in patient dissatisfaction and litigation.

Who, then, is the "ideal" candidate for aesthetic surgery? There is no such thing, but the surgeon should note any personality factors that will enhance the physical improvements sought. A person who has a clearly discernible physical problem about which he or she has an understandable, but not neurotic, concern is a good candidate. A person whose job requires him or her to look alert and well or who must compete with younger people is probably a good candidate. All these attributes are generally true, with the notable exception of the young male rhinoplasty patient—one who is single, immature, male, over-expectant, and narcissistic (S.I.M.O.N.). He is in a category by himself and should be evaluated with the utmost care. Generally speaking, men make more difficult patients than women. They do not tolerate pain as well and are generally more fussy.

There are basically two categories for rejection of a patient seeking aesthetic surgery. First is anatomic unsuitability. Second is emotional inadequacy. Since the latter is by far the more important, the inexperienced surgeon must learn to differentiate between healthy and unhealthy reasons for a patient's desire for aesthetic improvement. In the article following, we try to help you identify precisely the candidate for elective surgery who is not appropriate for selection.

AN OUNCE OF PREVENTION

There should be a frank discussion of fees and costs, if not by you, then by someone on your staff. Experience has shown that payment in full (and in advance) for cosmetic surgery diminishes subsequent unhappiness with final results.

It is far safer to accept a patient at the first visit. It is wise to ask him or her to think about what you have said, and return (at no fee). You should also ask the person to write down any questions, and at the second visit, go over the highlights of the original conversation and cover, once again, the most significant complications that may occur. Only when you are convinced that the patient is well motivated and understands what you have told him or her, you should allow surgery to be booked.

It is axiomatic that all patients undergoing surgery with local anesthesia be adequately sedated. No operative permit should be signed after sedation is administered as it may be held invalid. Every member of the surgical team should understand clearly that the patient, under the influence of narcotics, may misinterpret the most innocent words or jokes. Under no circumstances should there be arguments of any kind. There should be no swearing for any reason. Assistants and/or observers should be warned to save questions and comments for later. Finally, there is no such word as "*oops*" in the operating room; whether the surgeon drops a hemostat or comminutes the nasal bones, the word simply does not exist. It helps to talk to the patient and to be highly visible at the beginning and end of the procedure.

At the end of the operation, the surgeon should immediately report to the family. If no family members are present, a telephone call may be a very inexpensive investment. A visit to the patient on the evening of the operation is immensely reassuring. The surgeon should be the last face the patient sees before the anesthetic takes effect and the first one whom he or she focuses in the recovery room. Discharge instructions should be clear, specific, and in writing. Availability during the first few days is essential. If the surgeon signs out, it should be someone equally competent who takes charge, and the patient should be appraised in advance.

When dressings come off, there are innumerable questions, all of which require simple, reassuring answers. These questions will be fewer and less anxious if they have been answered preoperatively.

EFFECTIVE COMMUNICATION AS A CLAIMS-PREVENTION TECHNIQUE

All litigation in plastic surgery has a common denominator—poor communication. Underlying all dissatisfaction is a breakdown in the rapport between patient and surgeon. This vital relationship is often shattered by the surgeon's arrogance, hostility, coldness (real or imagined), and mostly the fact that "he or she didn't care." There are only two ways to avoid such a debacle: (1) make sure the patient has no reason to feel that way, and (2) avoid the patient who is going to feel that way no matter what is done.

Although the doctor's skill, reputation, and other intangible factors contribute to a patient's sense of confidence, a substantial part of what is called "rapport" between patient and doctor is based on forthright and accurate communication. It is faulty communication that most often leads to the inevitable vicious cycle that follows: disappointment, anger, or frustration on the part of the patient, reactive hostility, defensiveness, and arrogance from the doctor, deepening patient anger, and finally, a visit to the attorney.

Positive rapport can weather all sorts of treatment failures and complications. The art of good effective listening and speaking is rewarded by friendship, understanding, and good rapport. In the doctor-patient relationship, this interaction assumes critical importance, as the treatment outcome may literally depend on it.

ANGER: A ROOT CAUSE OF MALPRACTICE CLAIMS

As plastic surgeons, we tend to forget that medical litigation is inevitably a distillate of a simmering cauldron of emotional, psychological, and even psychiatric ingredients. All malpractice claims have anger as one of their root causes. It may be of the patient, it may be of the doctor, or it may be of both, but anger is always present. If we understand and learn to control this emotional aspect of medical misadventures, we can dramatically modify the outcome of an unfavorable result.

Virtually every patient contemplating medical treatment senses variable degrees of anxiety. From the surgeon, he or she also seeks reassurance against his or her uncertainties. An unfavorable outcome evokes feelings of despair and helplessness that may quickly turn to hostility. Regardless of the true cause of the result, such hostility will be focused on the most convenient and visible target: the doctor.

An unfavorable outcome also produces anxiety for the physician. More often than not, patient complaints are interpreted as personal affronts that strike the doctor's sense of professionalism, pride, and competence.

When the complaint is perceived by the doctor as being unwarranted, this complex human interaction may quickly degenerate into mutual hostility. A vicious cycle is then established: the physician's anxiety, guilt hostility, and arrogance are countered by hostility of the patient, and the physician's hostility mounts. In this climate, the possibility of a lawsuit quickly becomes a probability.

It is very difficult, if not impossible, to be objective when one is a party of an incipient lawsuit. Nonetheless, if it were possible to change the course of events prior to the onset of mutual hostility, the vast majority of malpractice actions could be avoided. The pretreatment or preoperative consultation, during which informed consent is obtained, can become a unique occasion for the doctor-patient relationship to be firmly established through the "sharing of uncertainty."

ACCURATE MEDICAL RECORDS: YOUR PRIMARY LINE OF DEFENSE

Regardless of its merits, any medical malpractice suit can be won or lost because of the quality and content of the medical records. Bear in mind that most suits are tried (or settled) years after the critical events. By that time, memory has faded, and the principal players may not even exist. In court, the records are the script by which the actors structure the play. The metaphor is uncomfortably close to the truth. Often what happens in the adjudication of a claim is much closer to drama than a search for truth. The actors with the best scripts win.

A suit of dubious merit can be lost because the medical record was vague, incomplete, and/or "added to." Conversely, a potentially damaging suit can be won because the medical record was thorough, accurate, and well-documented. The following guidelines summarize the simple requirements of a defensible record.

GENERAL GUIDELINES

1. The consequences of illegible handwriting can be costly. Be certain that your entries in all medical records are clear and readable. If possible, dictate all long entries that require more than brief or routine annotations.
2. Never "squeeze" words into a line or leave blank spaces of any sort. Draw diagonal lines through all blank spaces after an entry.
3. Never erase, overwrite, or try to ink out *any* entry. In case of error, draw a single line and write *error* with the date, time, and your initials in the margin.
4. Never *ever* add anything at any time unless it is in a separately dated and signed note. Remember that the entry date of ink or type can be accurately determined retrospectively. Also be aware that the plaintiff's attorney may have a copy of the patient's original records, and any alteration after the fact will seriously compromise the defense of your case.
5. The date and time of each entry may be critical. Be *sure* that each page is dated and bears the patient's name and that each progress note is accompanied by the date and time.

6. Avoid personal abbreviations, ditto marks, and initials. Use only standard and accepted medical abbreviations.

7. Retain your records for a minimum of 7 years from the date of the last entry.

The Patient's Records

The following entries should appear in the office and/or hospital records of each patient:

1. History and physical, specifically noting absence of abnormality.

2. Past history, with particular emphasis on current medications, allergies, drug sensitivities, or previous surgery.

3. Specific notation on the patient's experience, if any, with nicotine use, drug, or alcohol abuse, or previous surgeries.

4. Progress notes, entered after each office visit, on any change in status. If negative, your follow-up should be indicated.

5. Signed and witnessed consent forms for special procedures or surgery.

6. Medications, treatments, and specimens (where sent).

7. Patient's response to medications or procedures.

8. Document patient's failure to follow advice or to keep appointments, or refusal to cooperate; missed appointments should be logged. Record your follow-up telephone calls and letters.

9. All significant laboratory, pathology, and X-ray reports and the dates when ordered and read, the results acknowledged with the surgeon's initials and dated.

10. Copies or records of instructions of any kind (including diet) and directions to the family.

11. Consultations with other physicians and their written (or oral) responses with the date and time recorded.

12. Thorough documentation of any patient's grievance, including the date and time.

13. The critical importance of preoperative and postoperative photographs cannot be overemphasized. They should be of the same pose, lighting conditions, and quality; in plastic surgery claims, these photographs can literally spell the difference between the attorney's refusal to take the case or a substantial plaintiff's verdict.

SURGICAL CASE RECORDS

You should monitor the following reporting procedures to ensure that they are performed routinely:

Anesthesiologist

1. Accurate entries by the anesthesiologist, including type of monitoring device.
2. Condition of patient on transfer to recovery ward, including status of airway and position of the patient.
3. Post-anesthesia instructions signed by a responsible person on behalf of the patient.

Surgeon

1. Accurate operative notes of the surgeon dictated on the day of the procedure and including postoperative orders signed by the operating surgeon.
2. Postoperative instructions signed by a responsible person on behalf of the patient and acknowledged with their signature on the post operative record.
3. In outpatient cases, a notation by the surgeon of the patient's condition on discharge and when possible a record of a follow-up phone call on the evening of the surgery. (This is beneficial as much for documentation as for its rapport-building effect.)

Instructions

1. *Always* record your instructions in writing. Keep a copy in the patient's record.
2. Review your instructions with the patient and family.
3. Ensure comprehension. Ask and record if there are any questions after instructions.
4. Instructions should include (when applicable)
   a. Specific wound care.
   b. Limitations of activity, position, or exercise.
   c. Dietary restrictions.
   d. Specific instructions on medications, including possible side effects.
   e. Follow-up appointments.
5. Document
   a. Language limitations, attempts made to overcome them by translators, and your notation if comprehension appears to be questionable.
   b. Any literature provided to the patient and family, and/or video orientations.
   c. Copy of instructions given.
   d. Failure to comply with instruction, and that the patient was informed of risks of non-compliance.

CLAIMS PREVENTION IN OFFICE PROCEDURES

Not infrequently, the root cause of malpractice allegation is a series of events that begins with procedural errors in the office.

MISFILED REPORTS

One common practice that often leads to malpractice claims is the filing of reports that have not been seen by the doctor. This kind of carelessness can result in a delay in diagnosis or treatment of a serious disease. Laboratory, radiology, and pathology reports, X-rays, and consultation letters from other physicians should *never* be filed unless they have been seen and initialed by you.

PATIENT NON-COMPLIANCE

A situation that requires special procedures and attention relates to a patient's non-compliance or outright refusal to follow the doctor's order or recommendations. This problem may be more apparent to your staff than to you.

The staff should record missed appointments in the chart and call them to your attention. If the patient's non-compliance carries the potential for possible injury, a *certified* return-receipt letter expressing appropriate concerns for the patient's welfare and (when indicated) warnings regarding the consequences should be sent.

Suspense files should be set up for all tests, procedures, and consultations. If the tests are not carried out, the staff should call this to your attention, and the patient should be reminded. Patient non-compliance and callbacks to the patient should be recorded in the chart. Copies of all letters to the patient should be included.

In case of continued non-compliance and if circumstances warrant, a *certified* return-receipt letter also should indicate the withdrawal of your care. Notations of all actions and copies of all letters sent to the patient should become a permanent part of the patient's record.

INAPPROPRIATE BILLING

Another major factor that contributes to litigation is the continual billing of an already dissatisfied patient. If a dispute occurs, stop all billing action until it is resolved. Furthermore, if the patient has indicated dissatisfaction with a treatment or surgical procedure, consider forgiving the outstanding balance due.

The staff should promptly correct billing or collection errors and keep collections current to avoid a potential collision between the office staff and patients.

SPECIAL IDENTIFYING LABELS

Identify any drug allergies, and instruct the staff to display them prominently on a color coded label placed in a specific location on the outside of the patient's chart. Special labels also should be used for identifying nicotine users and if the case is a medico-legal or compensation case.

TELEPHONE ROUTINES WITH INSURANCE COMPANIES AND ATTORNEYS

The staff should not discuss the patient's medical problems or records without a release signed by the patient (or legal guardian) and the approval of the appropriate person in your office. The date, time, and name of the person calling and the purpose of the call should be recorded in the patient's chart. When requesting authorization from an insurance company to perform a treatment, tests, or other procedures, the staff must make sure that the patient has submitted a general release as a member of a plan. They should record the date, time, and name of the person authorizing the treatment, test, or procedure.

COMMUNICATION WITH PATIENTS IN THE OFFICE

Encourage your staff to initiate personal contact with patients by expressing warmth and individual attention. Impress on the staff that their conduct may represent the first, last, and most durable impression that patients have of your office and therefore of you. The staff can make it a favorable one by their demeanor.

INFORMING THE PATIENT

If you obtain the patient's consent, be sure that you have coordinated with your staff what you have told the patient so that your answers do not differ materially from one another. When performing any procedure on a patient, you should explain what is about to take place, and questions should be answered. Informed patients are much less anxious and much more cooperative. There is, for example, a substantial difference in reaction when you say, "This may hurt momentarily," than when you say, "This won't hurt at all," to a patient with a low pain threshold.

The staff should be familiar with legally required forms (such as breast cancer alternative treatment forms) and constraints in the treatment of minors or incompetent individuals.

AVOID MISTAKES

Double-check the vial or bottle prior to drawing up a substance. *Never* permit the existence of unlabeled vials or bottles in your operating room. If they are discovered, immediately discard them.

Make sure that your staff understand dosage: "15" or "50" may sound similar, but the difference may be catastrophic.

Prior to the administration of any medication by *any* route, the patient should be asked about allergy to the drug or drugs that are to be administered, even when there is no indication of drug allergy on the patient's chart.

Everyone should know the location and use of oxygen, crash cart, and other resuscitative equipment and drugs. Generally, the very first thing that should be considered in any untoward reaction is to start oxygen. If a staff member is along with the patient, he or she should maintain an open airway and call for help.

All personnel dealing directly with patients should be trained in cardiopulmonary resuscitation and should be recertified at appropriate intervals.

Develop with your staff guidelines for prescription calls and refills, and always record them with the date and time in the patient's chart.

EQUIPMENT MALFUNCTION

Most equipment-related suits involve electric burns. Be sure to check all electrical equipment to confirm that it is properly *grounded*.

A staff member should be assigned responsibility for ensuring that new personnel are instructed in the correct use and maintenance of all office and operating room equipment, and their initial utilization of the equipment should be supervised by an experienced person.

There should be a regular schedule of preventive maintenance. A bio-engineer should certify safety of electrical equipment on a regular basis. A log of such certification, with a reminder of the next scheduled service, must be maintained. A desirable place to keep the log is on a label affixed to the instrument itself.

The staff can make a vital contribution to achieving a pleasant, efficient office where very few mistakes occur and *preventable errors* are eliminated. Improved communications, procedures, administration, and system routines in a medical office and surgical suite are everyone's responsibility. The reward is that everyone benefits: the patient, the staff, and the physician.

CONCLUSION

It is simply not possible to summarize all you need to know into one chapter, or even into a whole book for that matter. It is also unrealistic for us to say, "This is what I do; if you follow our advice, you too can stay trouble-free." Unfortunately, it is not that simple. We have, therefore, tried to limit this chapter to principles and specific recommendations applicable to everyone. In the last analysis, though, even with strict adherence to these recommendations, there is no guarantee of an absolution, as we are dealing with intangible elements such as personality characteristics, ego structure, social conscience, and strong economic incentives.

It is not likely that in the coming decades there will be any major changes in our legal system. For this to happen, American jurisprudence would have to undergo revolutionary changes, and public morality a renaissance. Therefore, the next generation of plastic surgeons is plainly going to have to learn to live with the existing system of adjudicating medical injury. We have to develop the ability to change the things that we can, the serenity to accept those things which cannot be changed, and be wise enough to know the difference.

CHAPTER TWELVE

The Liability Carrier's Point of View

A plastic surgeon currently practicing in the United States may find it virtually impossible to end his or her career unblemished by a claim of malpractice. Recent changes to the liability climate may have reduced the frequency of claims filed against surgeons, but the severity of the final settlement or verdict amounts has actually increased. This means that when a claim does get filed, the financial consequences may still be significant. At the time of this writing, approximately two-thirds of the states have passed either some form of regulations positively affecting the malpractice insurance climate or significant tort reform including caps on noneconomic damages. Some of these changes have been challenged in the court system and have been modified or overturned as unconstitutional. But the ability of the malpractice carriers to reduce premiums based on a very real climate change in many states is for now a verified trend.

Despite these positive changes, however, it is still a fact that more than half of claims filed against plastic and reconstructive surgeons might have been preventable. With patient selection being an inexact science and surgeons facing complex psychological issues when determining who to operate on, the substitution of sound surgical decision-making for other motivations still occurs, especially when economic decisions overcome doing the right thing. Can this behavior be modified by decree or law or a well-intentioned malpractice insurance company? No. As a result, there will always be a need for malpractice insurance in the specialty of plastic surgery. The frequent claims filed because of dissatisfaction with the outcome, or the scar, will remain stable no matter how many states pass reforms. The fact that many of the so-called frivolous claims are eventually dropped, settled for reasonable amounts or won at trial, means the specialty is still considered a good risk when insurance business models are applied.

When plastic surgeons encounter the issue of malpractice insurance, it is most often at the time of purchase or payment for the policy itself. Until something goes wrong, there is rarely a need to have any further interactions with the carrier. But the other type of encounter, the need for claim management, is a serious matter that will mean getting to know several people employed by the insurance company. These relationships will, by necessity, need to be built rapidly, as responses to the initial legal filing by law cannot be ignored. Suddenly, the company who collected the payment and then disappeared from mind has become the most important conveyor of the surgeon's trust overnight. When everything is finally finished, relationships will remain that will be deep and emotional, like those of fellow combat veterans. The face of the company will go from an impersonal behemoth to that of a deeply personal and private trust peppered with very real people in the matter of a very short time.

Few surgeons spend much time investigating their malpractice insurance company. When the subject matter is insurance, the quickest decision is to shop price and local reputation. When a plastic surgeon joins an established group, there may not be any choice at all. The relationship with the company that covers the group may already be established, preventing any investigation into the matter.

The most common plastic surgery practice type however, solo, or solo in a shared office space, means that the malpractice decisions will be made by the surgeon alone, with the policy options reviewed only by himself or herself. Traditionally, the marketing of insurance policies to this surgeon has meant appealing to a single decision-maker, the selling points being more personal and individual. The issue then is truly one of relationships, with an insurance broker who then becomes the initial and perhaps the only face of the company (and may in fact be able to offer more than one choice and a range of products and different policies.) The skill of the surgeon to make a sound decision can at this point be totally dependent not on a relationship with the company *per se* but on the past experience with his or her own claims and that of a broker who understands this and can interpret the policy and the language therein. It is possible after this point that there will be few other personal interfaces the surgeon will have or need, perhaps until the first claim is filed. Hopefully, however, some other more personal interfaces with the company will occur such as attending a risk management seminar produced on a specific topic and offered to all policyholders, regardless of their claim history.

But what is the perspective from the other side? Are plastic surgeons just numbers, binary digits on a spreadsheet hidden away until something terrible happens? It is easy for the surgeon purchaser of a malpractice policy to feel that the behemoth company is impersonal, cold, and blithely ignorant of what he or she does in this unusual surgical specialty. After all, living without malpractice protection these days is virtually impossible, as to have hospital privileges means the surgeon is required annually to produce evidence of an up-to-date policy with limits on the amount of payment that will be made within the year and per claim. These limits are dictated either by the hospital or, in some instances, by the state statutes and regulations.

But to the surprise of many a plastic surgeon, liability insurance companies for the most part are actually very mindful of what this specialty is all about, as their financial success depends on avoiding large losses. As trends occur within the specialty for settlements and verdicts, the companies will adjust the premiums they charge to cover any such spike in payouts so that the risk is spread across the realm of policyholders. This is the reason for their existence, and to ignore changes in direction of the specialty would eventually mean losses that would catch up with the premiums charged–not a sound philosophy. But in a stable specialty and a stable environment, there is likewise a duty to the policyholders to reduce premiums whenever possible as well.

This assumes that all carriers are created equal. In fact, the majority of policies sold to plastic surgeons these days come from companies run by physicians or from a physician-owned mutual or reciprocal company. Only one-third of all physicians in the United States are covered by large carriers owned by shareholders rather than policyholders and specializing not only in liability policies but also in other lines of insurance. Many plastic surgeons find themselves in a program run by their state medical society and may know personally one or more of the elected board members, fellow physicians who have been involved in the medical society and visible for years to other colleagues. Here the risk is pooled amongst the many policyholders; premiums will still be based on the known risk for each specialty and the personal history of claims by each policyholder.

As the specialty of plastic surgery has a stable and easily determined history of risk, it is up to the carriers to determine if this market is right for them. For most companies, the answer has always been yes, especially because the reputation for plastic surgeons traditionally is for high frequency of claims but low payouts in the event of an unfavorable ending to the claim. Many claims filed against plastic surgeons can be categorized as "frivolous," inexpensive to manage, short in duration, and are either settled for a reasonable amount or are simply dropped when the plaintiff's attorney understands the strength of the defense team's position.

As a result, the companies who must calculate the costs they expect to encounter 3-5 years later must estimate with reasonable accuracy how much money to allocate for the actuality that a single large settlement or verdict could wipe out their reserves. In reality, state insurance regulations will prevent that from happening very often, but small carriers with risk spread across several hundred premiums instead of several thousand have been known to encounter one very large loss that eventually forced them into dangerous territory. For most companies then, spreading risk across plastic surgeons is a good alternative to other specialties such as neurosurgery or obstetrics where the settlements and verdicts can be disproportionately high if the case is lost.

THE COMPANY'S OBLIGATIONS TO THE SURGEON

Once the policy has been sold, the company owes both in principle and in writing some basic obligations to the surgeon. This includes acting in good faith when a claim has been made and making every effort to defend the claim the best it can. Financial protection for both the surgeon as well as the company becomes the primary goal. Surgeons expect that the company knows how to stay solvent. They also expect that, whether at settlement negotiations or at the trial, the company will do its best to keep any losses to within the stated limits of the policy, that is, to avoid financial ruin for the surgeon. The company also has the obligation to consider an appeal of any verdict for which there seems to be an unjust determination of the case.

The company is also obligated to provide legal representation in all claims brought about due to the medical actions of the policyholder. Each company will write specific portions of their policies to define exactly what it considers a covered action and what will not be covered. A patient, for example, tripping in the surgeon's waiting room and suffering a neck injury is not a covered act when he or she files suit against the surgeon for those injuries. Acts performed as an officer of the hospital usually are not covered under liability policies. Gray areas, such as offering Good Samaritan assistance in public to injured persons, may not be covered as well. Any advice or treatment in the emergency room, however, must be covered under the limits of the policy unless otherwise stated specifically. Each company will have developed specific portions of the policy to its own standards. These should be inspected closely from time to time by the surgeon to know exactly what is and what is not considered a covered event.

The company also has an obligation to stay solvent and maintain financial reserves to withstand high and unexpected losses. The policyholders assume that the money taken in through premiums will be enough to pay each year's verdicts, settlements and the costs of doing so, as well as the costs of keeping the company running. Beyond that, the company has no obligation to the surgeon in regard to its management of the reserves and investments, other than to have policies in place to avoid investment losses through high-risk behavior with those reserves.

When a surgeon retires, due to the protracted nature of filing a malpractice claim, he or she is not immune from the event that an unhappy patient decides to seek compensation several years later. The statute of limitations for each state will determine how much time must expire before any legal action against the surgeon is no longer binding; most states declare this limit to be 2-3 or 4 years. In some specialties such as pediatric surgery, the statute is exceedingly longer, up to age 18 for the patient.

Providing liability insurance until this time frame has been met is entitled "tail coverage." Anyone who has ever purchased a liability product will be familiar with the concept. The company will have an obligation when selling this policy to also state how much this rider to the end of the surgeon's practice will cost. It is not uncommon as an incentive to stay with the company to issue "free" tail coverage if the surgeon has bought yearly policies for, say, 5 years in a row. The decision, however, to purchase more than the usual tail coverage is up to the physician, but few surgeons ever retire without some form of added protection such as this.

Companies selling malpractice insurance are also obligated from time to time to periodically perform a review of the surgeons' practice through the underwriting department of that company. Such actions will provide an estimate of risk behavior found in the practice, allow calculation of the likelihood that this practice behavior will eventually result in an action against the policyholder, and allow adjustment of rates of the policy to reflect that. The obligation in this sense is actually to the other policyholders more so than the physician being reviewed, as it will even out the risk over all the policies, avoid an unexpected claim with high costs, and jettison policyholders deemed to be at high risk.

THE SURGEON'S OBLIGATIONS TO THE COMPANY

Once the policy has been sold, the company has most likely performed its analysis of the surgeon through its underwriting department. The decision to sell the policy will at that point be based on the surgeon's history of previous claims, the location and nature of the practice, and other information related to the odds of one day receiving a claim from a patient. The expectation is that the surgeon will continue to behave in a certain pattern and that altering by decree the surgeon's usual and customary practice behavior is an activity where the results will be rather limited.

There will be at times information sharing from the company to the policyholders, often in the form of risk management, such as publications offering advice or educational seminars that hopefully will make the surgeon aware of behaviors that can increase the likelihood of a claim and should be avoided. Beyond that, there is little else the company expects except for the following.

The surgeon policyholder has just a few obligations to the company issuing his or her malpractice policy. They will often be stated in writing within the policy and can include several important issues that require interaction with the company.

The most important of these is the timely reporting of an action against the surgeon. Once a patient has served notice of the intent to sue or serves the surgeon with a subpoena, the policy will require that the company be notified immediately of this action. In fact, most companies urge that policyholders inform them prior to the formal notice when there are multiple indications the patient intends to file suit. This notice serves to aid the company in setting aside reserves with the expectation they will be needed in the not too distant future. They will then also assign the problem to a claims manager, an employee experienced in this area and who becomes the intermediary between the physician, the patient, their attorney, and the company.

Some states require that a notice of intent to sue be sent to the surgeon in a specified time period prior to the actual filing of the legal paperwork. Ignoring this intent notice and failing to pass it on to the company can in fact become a breach of conduct that may or may not become an important issue later for both parties. The sooner the malpractice carrier knows of this intent, the sooner they can assign it to the correct professionals in the claims department.

Letters from patients making demands for refunds, or outright threats to sue if revisions are not performed for free, should be considered precursors to lawsuits as well. While there is usually nothing binding in the policy that specifies these be turned over to the company upon receipt, it makes good sense to notify the claims department of these situations as they assist the surgeon in working with the patient to find common ground. If a refund or return to the patient is determined to be the best course, it should always be accompanied by fully binding legal statements the patient must sign, that terminates their rights to seek further compensation. Can the physician obtain these by himself or herself? Yes, but the specific language in the document is better off written by a professional rather than anything the surgeon can concoct and that will have stood the test of time situations.

IMPLIED OBLIGATIONS

The surgeon will have responsibilities that will not be placed in writing but are expected of him or her as part of simply being a good physician and of sound mind and judgment. These cover several areas, including obtaining appropriate tests and consultations to make a correct working diagnosis. Other expectations include timely referrals when appropriate and review of any recommendations for treatment made by consultants. Finally, with surgeons it is expected that a thorough and timely chart will be maintained that reflects all aspects of the care of the patient.

The perfect chart from the malpractice carriers' point of view would be thoroughly legible, or at best contain all entries in typed format, with a logical sequence indicating the physician's examination and the reasons for the changes in care that will be recommended. The expectation is that any layperson in a jury box reading the entries could grasp this chart as a complete documentation of the treatment history. All tests that have been ordered will have the surgeon's initials and date as well as the time the surgeon reviewed the written results. Similarly, all consults obtained from outside sources should have been read and signed by the surgeon. Sections for the history and physical examination of the patient should be complete and reflect how the past history could impact the decision whether to operate on the patient or not in a timely fashion. The patient's allergies and medication history is expected to be complete, updated as needed, and easily accessible. Overall, the chart should reflect what transpired between the physician and his or her staff over the time span that the patient was treated. Billing records can be maintained in a separate section of the chart or totally separated electronically, as long as they can be retrieved easily as needed.

With the advent of the electronic medical record and eventually the stipulation that all records be electronically portable, these standards may be inescapable. Ending the dilemma of the physician with illegible handwriting will only help the defense of claims in the future, but for now this problem is still too often encountered by a malpractice company forced to defend the chart that is sloppy, with scribbled entries, and is overall poorly maintained. The insurance company cannot force the perfect chart on anyone, but it makes good sense in a specialty where claims still get filed frequently that the chart is always considered the first step in defending oneself against any type of claim.

It is also implied that all surgeons will obtain in writing an informed consent document prior to putting the knife to the skin or performing any other treatment. The reason for this is well outlined in other chapters in this book. What procedures need informed consent can be controversial. But, in general, if the treatment alters the epidermis, it may have risk. And certainly anything that alters the dermis or tissues below this level must be considered a procedure that requires informed consent.

PERSONAL COUNSEL

Even though the company will determine who is the best legal counsel to obtain for a surgeon faced with the early stages of a claim, these services will be contracted to outside law firms that the surgeon usually has the right to refuse. Once the surgeon is satisfied that the best fit for a defense counsel has been met, the work of defending the claim will begin, but if faced with trial, the company may or may not determine that additional legal representation may be needed such as in the form of a lawyer experienced in litigation at trial. At this point, the surgeon is better off not providing interference or his or her own personal preferences.

At the beginning of a claim, if the surgeon has had successful past personal experience with other attorneys, or if other defense attorneys are known to him or her through reputation, most companies will review the request and often grant that request if fees are reasonable and if that counsel has the appropriate skills for the challenges of the claim and is available in the time frame needed.

But in some instances, surgeons have gone one step further and hired their own separate counsel, an attorney whose fees will most likely not be met under the conditions of the malpractice policy. Does this make sense? Yes, under certain circumstances. Most often the interaction with one's own attorney is a check system to reassure the surgeon that the assigned attorney from the company is indeed doing his or her best to keep the optimal outcome in view and within reasonable time limits. But more importantly, in the event that a settlement offer is made which may in fact be unfavorable for the surgeon, rather than argue against it alone, the surgeon in this instance may be better off speaking and negotiating through the private counsel. This is especially true if that settlement may risk the surgeon's professional reputation and require financial payments over and above the limits of the policy. Personal and financial ruin may not seem to be the most important issue to the company when a large settlement is being considered, but it is the only issue the surgeon will be thinking of at that moment.

Do these situations arise? Unfortunately, yes. Each company will have its own policy on when to settle a claim it deems unwinnable in a court-room, or that will risk a higher jury verdict that the defendants are willing to accept. The best policy for a surgeon is one that states in writing that the final determination whether to press on or settle is the prerogative of the surgeon. Everyone in the liability insurance business and many surgeons themselves will have stories of a tough decision, the one that stopped the settlement, forced the claim all the way to a jury, and then was exonerated by a defense verdict. For each and every one of these, there are more stories that unfortunately went in the opposite direction. Juries are unpredictable except in some venues where it can be successfully anti-cipated that they will side with the plaintiff and deliver super large verdicts in almost every case.

These decisions can be some of the toughest issues a surgeon will ever have to deal with. Having one's own attorney for advice and counsel makes good sense unless the case is completely straightforward. These fees, how-ever, will be the responsibility of the surgeon and can add up over a 4-year or longer course to resolution. Many feel in the end it was worth it when it gave them peace of mind that the final decisions were achieved correctly.

CHAPTER THIRTEEN

The Dilemma of the Expert Witness

The hallways of medical conventions and meetings often resound with heated discussions on the role of the expert witness in medical malpractice trials. Specialty societies continue to demonstrate a growing interest in minimizing the influence of the "hired gun," the expert witness, who makes his or her opinion available as it suits the particular needs of the attorney in medical malpractice litigation. Much has been written about how to testify. However, little has been said about the most fundamental decision: to be or not to be a witness.

The sad fact is that no other country in the world tries medical lawsuits before a jury of lay people. In every other country, magistrates who preside over cases seek professional advice from a pool of medical experts attached to the court. An expert may be questioned by counsel but has no relationship to either side. In the American system, both sides recruit and pay their own expert witnesses. This arrangement transfers the adversarial relationship between both attorneys to the experts.

Our system does something else; it makes advocates of physicians who testify, making it difficult for them to remain objective. More importantly, the high expert witness fees being paid to some experts clearly have become incentives to testify, further clouding the witnesses' objectivity.

For the physician considering becoming an expert witness, a review of the medical record allows him or her to decide whether to accept or reject the assignment. If the invitation is from the defense team, and the case is truly defensible, the decision should be easy and the prospect appealing. After all, what doctor would not be pleased to help defend another physician?

Even if the case is seen as insupportable, a polite declination may produce disappointment but few, if any, bruised egos.

An invitation to act as an expert witness for the plaintiff brings an array of totally unfamiliar exposures for the physician. Plaintiffs' attorneys will say they do not understand why doctors should have any conflict with testifying in court, much less emotional distress. To them an accusation of malpractice is routine, everyday business. They say, "It does not mean you are a bad doctor; it just means that you made a mistake. There is no need to get emotional about it!"

This attitude reflects total disregard for the effect of a malpractice allegation (win or lose, guilty or not) on a physician's perception of his or her competence, integrity, self-confidence, and values.

By the same token, peer approval holds a very high priority among our colleagues. Our psychological defense mechanisms also block us from accepting that our professional behavior, in any given instance, might have been less than stellar. This defensive reaction is coupled with the conviction that anyone who helps the plaintiffs' team has just bought a ticket to hell. Worse yet, the action is viewed as a knife in the back when it involves a colleague of the same specialty.

The nature of the ethical and moral dilemma facing expert witnesses is multifaceted and complex. Suppose the medical records show that the treatment was clearly inappropriate, and its direct result was serious, disfiguring, or life-threatening. Worse yet, suppose one knows that this surgeon had experienced a similar outcome in more than one case. What looms higher in one's conscience: obeying one's instincts or being totally devoted to the specialty and the image one might wish to have among those peers? Is the latter more important than the prevention of severe damage to an unlucky future patient? There is a vast difference between testifying in cases where the issue in question is the result of an inherent risk, unexpected complications, or just plain incompetence.

How does the surgeon expert testify against someone known in the community to be unscrupulous or incompetent? Can one be sure to always identify the sharp, bright line that defines those parameters?

A rational physician knows that medicine is an inexact art. Few would argue that compensation should be due to patients injured by probable negligence. What should be deplored are the glaring abuses that occur in the American way of resolving medical disputes. Similarly deplorable is that "acts of God" are often interpreted as liability in the American tort system.

Nonetheless, until the unlikely day when our tort system changes, we need to accept that ours is a truly adversarial one. We must also accept the responsibility of participating in our judicial system with as much integrity as our conscience can muster.

Physicians who testify for the defense are also obligated to ascertain that whatever actions the defendant chose to take were within the standard of care and that the results were totally beyond human control. Additionally, whatever the expert witnesses' testimony will be, that surgeon should be sure to have never held a contrary position to the one he or she is expressing now, either in an article, or worse yet, a different case from the past that slipped the mind. If opposing counsel then leads the expert witness down the primrose path and then surprises them with printed evidence of a contrary opinion, that surgeon might just as well pack his or her things and go home. Furthermore, they may also have torpedoed the side they were trying to help.

Plastic surgeons asked to act as the plaintiff's witness need not automatically refuse to participate as witnesses out of fear of besmirching their reputations. This responsibility, however, assumes a different priority: to separate fact from fiction, to know with certainty that the damage is one that was plainly outside the standard of care and to consider all extenuating circumstances.

Most importantly, the expert must consider whether the same event might have occurred had the case been under his or her own control. Then, and only then, can the surgeons decide in the loneliness of their mind whether the totality of the situation outweighs the constraints of the heart.

Prior to giving testimony at trial, the expert most likely will have been questioned by the opposing counsel in a deposition. Both before the deposition and after it, he or she will have had an opportunity to consult with the attorney who retained them, learned his or her views of the case, and heard suggestions and admonitions regarding the appropriate manner of testifying. The deposition testimony about to be given will be compared with similar testimony at trial, so before entering the courtroom, the expert witness must always be completely familiar with the transcript of the deposition.

If this is the first time to testify as an expert witness, one might be helped by arranging a visit to an empty courtroom. Before the trial proceedings, get a detailed explanation from the attorney about the "players," and the order of the procedure, that is, who is going to do what, to whom, when, and why. The attorney will also be the best advisor regarding details of proper decorum and courtroom caveats.

Respect the advice given by the attorney on one's side. This advice does not mean intervention in the substance of the expert's testimony but, rather, guidance about how to comport oneself and how to recognize a priori the techniques that the opposition is likely to use to devalue or mystify the upcoming testimony. There is an art to testifying and experienced attorneys can be of great assistance if one lets them.

The importance of the expert's demeanor from the moment he or she enters the courtroom until the testifying is finished cannot be exaggerated. Self-control, honesty, courteousness, and politeness are crucial elements to the success of this case, as is the wearing of appropriate attire. The latter, believe it or not, is a very important expression of the expert's professionalism which the jury is apt to notice. Jurors expect an expert witness to appear professional and serious. How one appears as well as what he or she says can send a very strong message about credibility and trustworthiness.

It is the expert's distinct advantage to understand that the judge is the absolute ruler in the realm of the trial and will tolerate no nonsense. Stepping into the witness stand should never include attempts to ingratiate oneself with familiarity or small talk. A nod and a smile are sufficient.

The expert's testimony will initially be to questions posed by the attorney who retained them. This is known as direct testimony. The attorney will always ask questions he or she has covered prior to the day in court, questions he or she hopes the answers to which will settle what is needed to be accomplished for his or her side. When the direct examination is finished, the opposing counsel will cross-examine the witness. This is the time one will need to maintain his or her confidence and cool.

Keeping one's demeanor and temper under absolute control at all times is critical, no matter what the circumstances. This is not an option; it is the very heart of a successful session on the stand. If self-control is sabotaged successfully by the other side deliberately for the purpose of "getting one's goat" (depending on the tactic being tried), it may be a turning point of the case in their favor. Humor, no matter how well intentioned, is not advisable and almost always falls flat. The best experts find other ways to cope with their nerves.

Attorneys will always advise the expert to give polite but firm answers to questions asked and to restrain from digressing. One should never offer spontaneous information. Any uncertainty about issues in the case should have been discussed with the attorney prior to trial, to the satisfaction of both parties. Questions one can't then answer should be handled as such. Much more damage can be done inadvertently to the cause when an uncertain answer is given than when the expert simply states "I don't know the answer to that question." The expert's responses should never be given in a tone of arrogance as both judge and jury will sense it and view it negatively.

It is important to speak slowly, authoritatively, clearly, and audibly. Pause before answering questions. Do not blurt out a thing. When one does not understand a question, or even if one is just stalling for time, the expert should never be afraid to ask for a repetition of the question or an explanation.

Be on the alert for deliberate obfuscation by the interrogator. It should not be difficult in most instances to sense where he or she is going with the line of question, thus, one can be prepared to avoid or at least defuse the climax with a gently phrased response. It will not go unnoticed. Very frequently, lawyers cleverly arrange a string of questions so that they can trap a witness at the end with a demand for a "yes" or "no" answer. This will be posed in such a way to guarantee that one's response will be detrimental to the case. Because in medicine there are seldom purely black or white answers, it is not out of order for an expert to reply by stating precisely that. But some alternative answer should be entertained as well, if needed. If the badgering continues, a good expert witness might certainly turn to the presiding judge and explain the difficulty of answering yes or no to a "maybe" question. At that point, however, a good attorney will probably have intervened with an objection anyway. Whatever happens, once again, the best experts always will keep their composure and remember that these kinds of tactics seldom sit well with the jury.

Every trial lawyer has his or her own bag of tricks; some subtle, some blatantly obvious. Watch for them. Sometimes, they may take the form of a less than flattering comment or a humorous remark about doctors or the practice of medicine that is intended to distract the expert's focus. The most effective response should be that one has been taught since childhood never to denigrate anyone's occupation. Resist the temptation to add, "...even a trial lawyer." The questioner will regret having made the comment and the jury will take note.

It is, by now, ancient pre-trial advice that when answering questions on the witness stand, the best witness will speak in the direction of the jury. The best analogy of an effective expert witness' style of testifying is that of a teacher. The jurors need to learn about a subject that is largely foreign to them; they are looking to the expert for assistance.

It is natural to focus one's attention on those who are concentrating seriously on what is going on and whose emotions are discernable by facial expression. Cynics say that if a witness gets good at this, he or she can at least firmly convince one or two jurors to stay on his or her side no matter what. If things go awry, then the very worst outcome might be a hung jury. On the other hand, none of what is said or not said should be mistaken as currying favor with any of them.

During direct testimony, it is extremely useful to have a marking board and colored chalk in the courtroom. The attorney may have you use it in your effort to "teach" the jury, so be sure that the equipment is there. The work of a plastic surgeon, more than any other physician, is easy to explain with diagrams. Don't get too esoteric. Simply clarify what you want the judge and jury to understand and stay away from medical terminology as much as possible. You will not only impress the jury, but also will leave them with a much clearer comprehension of your testimony.

In a medical liability trial, certain generic questions specifically designed to put you in a bad light frequently emerge. It pays to have a prepared response which goes beyond a "yes" or "no" answer. For example:

Q: Doctor, how much are you getting paid to come here and testify against my client?

A: I will submit a fee for my appearance here, not because I am testifying but only for the time here that prevents me from attending to my patients and my practice.

If the attorney persists, provide an hourly figure rather than a lump sum. It will not sit well with the jury if you are badgered, but they also won't like it if you are obviously dodging the question.

Q: Doctor, are you familiar with Dr. Plastikos and/or his popular text (articles) on Transplantation of the Head, research that is familiar to most surgeons?

A: I am.

Q: What is your opinion of his work?

A: All of us admire and respect Dr. Plastikos for his innovative work and know him to be a highly regarded teacher. However, those of us in active practice also know that in our line of work some procedures become the standard of care for a period of time, then evolve or are superseded later by newer and better techniques. Dr. Plastikos may have even changed his thoughts by now as the publication you refer to is now X years old. Plastic surgery is a continually evolving art and the most challenging aspect of our craft is that there are normally several different techniques within the standard of care that achieve the same level of excellence. In plastic surgery, "different" doesn't equate with "bad" if the end result is the same.

Whatever one may personally think of the defendant or the opposing expert, it reflects poorly on one's case to denigrate any colleague overtly or by implication for any reason. It will be a black mark against the expert's testimony. By the same token, if it is the honest opinion that an avoidable error has been made, then as the expert witness, you are bound by your oath and integrity to say so, always, of course, with prior consultation with the attorney and with the least prejudicial language one can muster.

Invariably, in cases involving plastic and reconstructive surgery, the issue of books and journals comes up. The expert will almost surely be asked what professional reading he or she "keeps up with." In addition to whatever medical literature is cited, the expert should be prepared to point out that regardless of topic, all medical texts have a limited time span in which the information remains valid. It is only a matter of the passage of time for any reference to lose its value. If either the defendant or opposing witness happens to be the author who has been published, it is a sure thing that the other side will have read every single word he or she has ever written. It is recommended that one would do likewise before coming to court to avoid stammering foolishly in the witness stand. If it is a book chapter, article, or quotation that is at issue, there will probably be a lively discussion as to its accuracy and its relativity to current treatment and standard of care.

If the matter of flexibility in choosing how to treat is at issue, consider emphasizing one's point by citing examples such as the following:

1. Skin cancer can be just as effectively treated by direct excision, by flap, by skin graft, or even by radiation, depending on a number of factors. There is no inflexible code.

2. Breast hypertrophy can be treated by several techniques with equally good results, again depending on a number of factors. However, at no time does the description of any operation in the medical literature constitute a definitive treatment or one that indicates a permanent standard of care because of the evolutionary nature of plastic surgery technology.

In conclusion, it must be said that any service as an expert witness should be based on the desire to do what is right, not tailoring one's testimony to satisfy the highest bidder. I plead with my colleagues not to stride into the courtroom clad in the armor of a medieval gladiator but to serve humbly and honorably. Analyze the case carefully and be prepared to explain to the jury in accurate and understandable terms whether the injury was the result of inherent risk, unexpected complications, or incompetence. You can be sure that the opposing witness will rebut this testimony, so the better prepared one is and the more one understands the nature of the courtroom theater, the most likely the case will be judged in the expert's favor.

In all cases, by following the motto, "Thou shalt not bear false witness," the expert witness should be able to leave the witness stand with the respect of everyone in the courtroom and, most importantly, respect for oneself.

CHAPTER FOURTEEN

Coping with Bad News

The defining moment in the course of a claim against a plastic surgeon is the exact point in time when it can no longer be denied that the patient is indeed going to seek a malpractice suit. It is that instant when the summons, the ultimate engagement announcement, arrives blaring the truth. Quiet defiance at that point can no longer be the working paradigm. In fact, the delivery of bad news should not really be a shock at all, as the potential threat of an action by all indications should have been known or at least suspected. When angry patients make exacting demands for refunds, when unknown attorneys request copies of a patient's chart, when the office staff tip toes around the issue, only an imperceptive myopic surgeon should be shocked at this point to learn the truth. Disappointed? Yes. Stunned? Probably. Surprised? No.

The delivery of a summons at the doorstep, while it is the end of the suspense, is also the admission that a long journey has just begun. The gates are open and the horses have begun the race.

Throughout this book, we have assumed that up to this point all efforts to avoid claims have been adhered to; all the charting is perfect, the patient selection admirable, and the surgery carried out with skill and success. No matter what, the fact that a claim is indeed now coming forward reveals that what was hoped for can no longer be denied.

Nearly all surgeons eventually get sued. Those who don't during a protracted career are rare, or simply not doing much surgery at all. Nevertheless, when all control is lost and the threat becomes real, there are a new set of rules to live by and coping with them requires skills applied in ways that may not come naturally to all. In effect, this moment, while it should not spell defeat, will simply demand an admission that despite the surgeon's best efforts, no matter what took place before, there are now implications that will impact the self esteem, the lifestyle, and the practice, possibly for years.

The delivery of the summons by a process server can be thoroughly traumatic especially if it takes place at home on the doorstep, at the office waiting room, or the parking garage at the hospital. It is difficult to believe that this person dropping an envelope into your hands has a conscience and enjoys making a living by these acts. (Actually, such persons take this business seriously, as at times it requires sleuth-like skill, and they all have stories to tell.) But that said, what happens next is not pretty. A Pandora's box of emotions can be triggered by this weird and unusual event; some surgeons have likened it to an out-of-body experience.

What's worse is the initial reading of the complaint once the envelope is opened. Only a rare surgeon can examine the charges against him or her (and often the spouse) and not be personally traumatized by them. They will point out in specific terms how profoundly ignorant and unskilled the surgeon was, how the actions of the surgeon caused irreparable harm, and that it was all with intention and recklessness. It is difficult not to take this personally and to realize this is just part of the process; someone was just doing his or her job. In the haze and fog of what happens next, mistakes in judgment can be forgiven as emotions run wild.

Many surgeons report feelings of guilt, shame, resentment, and indignation at this point. That this is all terrifying is inevitable and to be expected. How one goes about dealing with those feelings, especially over the two to three or four year life span of the claim is critical. It should come as no surprise that many who have been forced to chart these waters have been diagnosed with stress related medical conditions such as cardiac conditions of all sorts, gastric ulcers, and depression. There will be a whole new set of rules to deal with, starting soon after this moment. Spelling out how they can affect every part of the surgeon's world is what we are concerned with here.

After the surgeon recovers from the initial impingement of his or her sense of honor, code of personal conduct and ethics, there are a number of things that must be done and in an orderly fashion. Above all else, this is the time to get to know the malpractice experts of one's insurance company on a personal level. Notifying them of what has happened soon after does two things: it provides professional help in dealing with the issues at hand and gives the surgeon an action plan.

Shortly after that, the chart will be the most prominent issue. From this point on, it cannot be altered as the copy that was sent to the attorney will at some point be compared to the original in the surgeon's possession. Making a number of copies, then locking up the original is what most surgeons are told to do, along with the caveat to in no way alter the record. No one on the surgeon's staff should have access to the original without the surgeon's permission and it must be in his or her control so that it cannot be inadvertently lost or damaged from its original state.

Next will be the first meeting with the claims manager assigned from the staff at the liability carrier and this should take place in a matter of days or a week or two, not months. This person is experienced in this arena and will get help with many of the questions and concerns surgeons will have at this point. He or she can be one's new best friend, is on the surgeon's side no matter what, and will set all the wheels in motion to reassure him or her that everything will be done in the surgeon's best interest. If this has not happened by the second or third meeting, one may wish to suggest that a different staff member be assigned to this claim, a prerogative not often realized, and rarely needed.

Initially, doubting this person's skill and experience is a common reaction. After all, he or she is not a surgeon, perhaps he or she does not have a clear understanding of the surgery one performs, and his or her initial questioning may be disquieting. As time wears on, however, this person will become a confidant like no other and will have a strong relationship with the attorney who eventually will handle the case. Landing a team of both a smart claims manager and a skilled defense attorney that has worked together successfully in the past is a godsend as each will know what the other can and will do.

As far as the choice of the attorney goes, unless the surgeon has a preference, the carrier will decide who best fits the unique problems in this case and who has the best defense record in surgical claims. But the surgeon should always have the last say. Knowing that a certain attorney successfully defended one's friends at the hospital is a terrific advantage, but surgeons should not take it personally when that superstar is too booked to even meet with him or her, or if the attorney becomes uninterested after hearing the facts of one's particular case. Enquire quietly who else has salvaged one's colleagues' cases and choose another one. In the end, one might be better off with the attorney the liability carrier wants to use and who should know better after all.

By now, the claims manager will also have asked the surgeon to put everything he or she can remember down on paper. This document, a running narrative of the case, will be protected under attorney-client privileges and will not be available to the plaintiff's counsel at any point. Writing things down often will stimulate memories of important moments in the case, what was said, what the staff might have recalled, and other details that never made it to the chart. The act of condensing this into a working document can also be cathartic, releasing emotions, and setting the resolve to win the case. Putting aside the time to get this right is important, and whether it takes a weekend or a few weeks more, it should be considered a first priority. It can be modified later but the claims manager will want to use it to formulate additional questions for the surgeon to answer. By now the defense of this claim should be shaping up.

It is at this point, however, that this chapter leaves the legal arena and goes to the heart. All of the above steps are well outlined in many articles and publications dealing precisely with the start of a lawsuit. Few of these, however, delve into the emotional torrent of feelings that become unleashed with the summons, and which can sweep the unsettled surgeon away in a river of self-doubt, anguish, and physical maladies.

The most difficult thing that surgeons must deal with after getting the defense team up and running is the admonishment that they should not speak to anyone about the facts of the case. Really? No one? No matter how cruel this may seem, there is logic in it and it must be dealt with honestly from this point on.

The first few questions that a surgeon faces at the deposition called by the plaintiff's attorney will include the simple inquest, "With whom have you spoken about this?" The answer and the way it is delivered will frame the next fifteen minutes to an hour or more of the deposition and give him or her a chance to make the surgeon seem a liar, lacking truth and ethics, and marking him or her immediately to be a dupe for the rest of the deposition.

Remember that one has just pledged to tell the truth, the whole truth, and nothing but the truth. It is a lot easier at this point to clearly answer "No one besides my attorney and my claims manager." Mention anyone else and there is always the threat that he or she will be subpoenaed and dragged into the battle as to what it was you said and when you said it. Lie at one's peril, but skilled attorneys can spot the truth and its ugly cousin, perjury, across the room. The surgeon's credibility as a witness may be lost on the first question. Being able to tell the truth is important.

But too often the mistake is made when this admonishment is taken too seriously. We are social animals and we advance our feelings daily through speech. How can one maintain sanity and talk to no one about what you are experiencing? This is precisely the trap that surgeons fall into when told they should not discuss this case with anyone.

Surgeons can however talk about their feelings and emotions, the ones that are so unsettling when facing a malpractice suit. Without revealing the details of the case, the specifics or even the outline of the case, they can freely discuss what the stress of this is doing to them, their marriage, their practice, and their health. Once this concept is understood, the defendant can realize that opening up about the weight of the experience with a trusted cohort is one of the best things that can be done toward making the entire ordeal livable.

Who to trust varies depending on the history and importance of past relationships. Sometimes, another surgeon who has a similar experience makes a great listener. Perhaps it is a priest, a rabbi, or a minster. Siblings, old friends, or neighbors can be trusted at times to listen, offer advice, and keep the consultations to themselves as well. Whoever fills this role becomes part of the team, invested in the process and hopeful of the best outcome. Their importance to the defendant sometimes parallels that of a spouse. In fact, in many cases surgeons wishing not to overburden their relationship with the spouse have found that the cohort relationship can actually help a marriage by taking the burden off the spouse to fulfill multiple roles.

There may, however, be times when unburdening oneself through dialogue just isn't enough. Sleep deprivation, constant anxiety over the personal and financial implications of losing the case, and the inability to concentrate about anything else may indicate that professional assistance is needed. Having one or two vegetative signs of depression is not uncommon when undergoing a protracted lawsuit. Loss of appetite, excessive worry, and frequent bursts of anger mean that it might be time to consider, at the least, taking an antidepressant, and maybe getting professional therapy. This is not an admission of weakness, though surgeons may feel at this point that they have succumbed to outside forces beyond their control. Prolonging much-needed treatment in instances such as this can compound the problems and amplify the entire situation. The positive effects certainly can outweigh the negative stigma when relations improve with the spouse, the family, the office staff, and patients.

Other positive steps include reducing the workload at the office, increasing exercise sessions, and taking more time off for therapeutic activities. Many surgeons feel that the two-to-three year ordeal prevented them from taking more personal time away from the office when in fact getting away may be just the thing needed to put some distance from the process. While it may take the first few days of a vacation to stop thinking about the claim and its developments and possible endpoints, the effects of the rest and relaxation when returning to it all can have dramatic changes on the overall perception of the claim progression.

Some surgeons feel that keeping a journal through the ordeal has helped them better understand their feelings and sentiments. It can have particularly gratifying effects when it is re-read at times and reveals that true emotional progress has taken place in the months and years that this goes on. Is it discoverable? The best answer is to share it with one's attorney at times so that it becomes part of the work product considered off limits under the attorney-client privilege.

In the end, there are some common mistakes that surgeons make when confronting a multi-year progression from claim to trial. Trying to prevent the spouse from going through the agony of the process and the day-to-day details can have a more negative impact on the marriage than the opposite effect. Assuming he or she should not have to share the anxiety means the potential loss of one more person to offer advice and commiseration. Surgeons sometimes feel that avoiding the assumed extension of their grief on others avoids the pity that might be expressed when what they really need is strength. Each relationship differs, but in the end the spouse can have significant positive effects on the surgeon's attitude and adjustment.

Another common problem is the failure to assess the bitterness and acrimonious feelings that come naturally toward the former patient. Facing down that person in deposition (if he or she attends) or finally in the courtroom can lead to explosive, if not rancorous, reactions. Admitting that there is a potential for this ahead of time and then planning how to deal with it can reduce the irrational and indignant feelings that will possibly surface at the moment one faces the former patient for the first time in years.

Lastly, most surgeons continue to practice, as they must during this lengthy process, no matter at what speed. The vast majority of the patients, if they knew about the surgeon's ordeal, would offer enormous levels of support. Of course, they cannot be told about it. (Only in rare cases does it become public knowledge through the press, and then the surgeon can only accept their support holding the line not to discuss the facts of the case with anyone.) But taking whatever strokes one can from happy patients is still critically important to the self-image and the ego at this point. What at one time may have been just another thank you from a satisfied patient takes on a whole new meaning in the context of enduring a lawsuit. Failing to understand the impact this can and must have is a real loss, one any surgeon should not have to work at to understand its value.

Winning the case will spell relief. Losing it will eventually bring an end to the nightmare and liberation in its own way. Whatever the outcome, it is more about how the surgeon plays the game than the final dispensation. Surviving the ordeal with an intact marriage, a normal level of self esteem, and a practice ready for the next level of success requires insight and skill. The suffering eventually disappears, the torment fades, and the nightmare pales away. The long view many years later will be significantly impacted by having the right attitude and awareness of the process, one we hope has become easier through our efforts at writing this book.

INDEX

Note: Page numbers followed by *f* indicate figures and *t* indicate tables